W9-BBY-263

BODY RESTORATION

- AN OWNER'S MANUAL

Michael Lebowitz D.C.

Ami Kapadia M.D.

www.bodyrestorationanownersmanual.com

Copyright © 2011 Lebowitz/Kapadia

All rights reserved.

ISBN: 146100294X
ISBN-13: 978-1461002949

DISCLAIMER:

The information in this book is based on the authors' clinical experience and contains the opinions and ideas of the authors. This book is not intended as medical advice, but is rather for educational and informational purposes only. While the information can be useful as a self-help guide, please seek the care of a medical or health professional if needed/indicated. The authors and publishers cannot take the medical or legal responsibility of having the information in this book considered as a treatment plan for everyone. Either you and/or your treating physician will be responsible for any recommendations that you implement from this book. Do not make any changes to prescription medications without consulting a physician.

The authors and publisher specifically disclaim all responsibility for any liability, loss or risk, personal or otherwise, that is incurred as a consequence, directly or indirectly, of the use and application of the contents of this book.

Table of Contents

INTRODUCTION

This book has been a long time in the making. I grew up with pollen and mold allergies, resulting in 13 years of weekly allergy shots that did very little to help the symptoms. Frequent stomach aches and headaches accompanied the allergies. As I grew older, the symptoms continued and, after moving to a mold infested house in rural West Virginia, I developed chronic fatigue with severe brain fog. After a car accident in 1980 and having my amalgams removed, I developed severe memory loss, mood swings and MS type numbness (I attribute most if not all of it to the mercury exposure during amalgam removal). This led me on a quest to many types of health care practitioners, and finally through my own research and my work in Applied Kinesiology, to develop some tools that have helped restore much of my health. I began attracting patients with similar symptoms plus a myriad of others. Despite living in a rural area, and with absolutely no advertising, I was being contacted by people from around the world seeking help. My perfectionism, prayer, and an unending desire to help these people over my 30+ years in practice have helped me to understand many of the underlying causes and how to correct them, if possible.

In 1984 I self published a book entitled *BODY MECHANICS- A guide to understanding and correcting Body Dysfunction at home.* Within a few years, it was sold out and out of print (though occasionally you can find a used copy online). I was asked to republish it, but due to a busy practice, young children at home, and other commitments, it was placed on the back burner. Every now and then my wife would keep encouraging me to put it back in print, but other than occasionally using it to teach a group of homeschoolers and their parents how to live a healthy life, I resisted.

In my practice, I began to realize the role that subclinical infections of various fungi, viruses, bacteria and parasites played in the health of so many of us and continue to do so at epidemic rates. I began to research the role of toxic chemicals and metals in health and disease as well as that of food sensitivities/toxins/allergies. I found that, in a majority of patients, if I could get rid of dysbiosis (chronic subclinical infections), figure out which foods they were sensitive to, detoxify the toxic metals and chemicals in their bodies, and replenish the nutrients they were deficient in, the patients would often get well. This was without addressing organ dysfunction because, in most cases, these above mentioned factors were the underlying cause of the organ dysfunction in the first place. This was one of the reasons *Body Mechanics* was not republished- I felt that unless I included this new information, the book would be missing many key concepts.

I began to develop techniques utilizing Applied Kinesiology, taking a detailed patient history concerning causative factors, and being an environmental and food detective for my patients. These techniques greatly helped many of my chronic patients and I began to teach them to other natural health care practitioners and have now done so for over 20 years. I also began a free monthly newsletter for health care professionals to share what I was learning (you can view back issues of it on my website www.michaellebowitzdc.com). This newsletter is now in its 22nd year and goes to almost 2,000 practitioners worldwide.

For the past year, I have had the valuable assistance of a colleague, Ami Kapadia MD, to help me in my practice and help consolidate some of my ideas. With my wife's challenge, we decided to take on the rewriting of *Body Mechanics*- updating the old information if needed and adding the necessary information on subclinical infections, toxic metals, food intolerances, etc., as well as supplements we have found to be incredibly useful. We have renamed the book *Body Restoration- An Owners' Manual.* We want it to serve a number of purposes:

1) Be a book the natural health care practitioner could give to his/her patient to help educate them in anatomy, physiology, and how various foods, microbes and toxins affect the body.

2) Be something a family could use to help them help themselves with more simple health issues and to complement the instructions of their physicians.

3) Act as a basic anatomy/physiology text for lay people in general with practical information on how to stay healthy or become healthier than you are at present.

4) Be educational for the health care practitioner not schooled in natural remedies, giving them another way to look at health and disease

Our bodies are a marvelous creation. The 21st century is very challenging for these amazing machines. We are bombarded by polluted air and water, toxic chemicals and metals, hybridized and genetically modified foods, increased mold and fungi levels in our air tight houses, electromagnetic fields from our computers, cell phones, wi-fi, etc. We are human guinea pigs in this high-tech environment, and it takes knowledge and work for many of us to stay well. We hope the ideas in this book can help in this endeavor.

Like *Body Mechanics,* we have a chapter on most organs with basic anatomy and physiology, causes of organ dysfunction (beyond just genetics which is always an unspoken factor), symptoms, prevention and treatment. We have also listed the supplements we find most useful. Most people will not need to take all the supplements but with patient experimentation, and hopefully the guidance of an alternative medicine practitioner, you can find which of these may work for you. There is also a separate chapter on supplements in the back that explains why we use the brands recommended in this book. Part 2 will discuss some of the most important underlying causes of illness: subclinical infections, toxins and food reactions. Understanding these and treating them are critical in health restoration.

Without the help of my wife Cynthia, who is more indispensable than she'll ever know, Dr. Kapadia, my sons (one of whom insists I am too lazy), my teaching partners over the years, my AK colleagues who continually share their ideas with me, and my patients, who I am always learning from, and many others- this book would not have all the information it presently has. I thank all of you for your contribution. I also thank Dr. Natalie Phelps, who has treated me with many of these techniques over the years.

I suggest you read the book cover to cover the first time through and then go back to various sections as a reference later. Don't let the technical terms deter you, as you will learn much and gain many practical tools to restore your health. Some sections build on others so reading it straight through is the ideal way to get the maximum benefit out of it.

This book will be accompanied (check for availability) by the *Body Restoration Cookbook* which has many recipes and ideas for people who do not tolerate nightshades, gluten, dairy, refined sugar, eggs, etc.

At www.bodyrestorationanownersmanual.com we will try to post helpful articles and updates. Physicians who want to learn advanced techniques can read about our DVD on the website: www.michaellebowitzdc.com

May God guide you,

Michael Lebowitz DC

From my earliest exposures to health care, I have been drawn to a more natural way of healing rather than relying on quick-fixes and pharmaceuticals. Although I am still early in my career, I have had the opportunity to learn from some truly inspirational integrative medicine practitioners who showed me a different way to approach health and illness. The concept of functional medicine and its guiding framework in addressing almost all symptoms and illnesses has been key in my personal development of the knowledge to help people beyond superficial symptom based prescriptions. While I believe allopathic medicine has a definite role in certain situations, I find that it often fails in adequately treating chronic illness. By addressing the key "root causes of illness" discussed in the second half of this book, I believe many patients can start to understand the factors that can lead to "disease" and dysfunction, and how addressing them can help to restore function and reduce symptoms through a natural approach.

My own personal health challenges motivated me to seek alternative solutions to allopathic medicine. Starting over a decade ago, I began to suffer from severe headaches/migraines, among other symptoms. After seeing some of the best specialists that traditional medicine could offer, I had at times lost hope for recovery and a normal life. For several years, my quality of life was severely affected, and my daily activities consisted of just trying to "get through the day." It became difficult to make plans as I had no idea how I would feel from one day to the next, and when the next severe headache would strike. I was fortunate enough to gain exposure to integrative medicine through a physician that became one of my mentors in medical school. As I sat in with him, and other practitioners in our community, I learned of new concepts such as dysbiosis and toxicity. I soon realized how my diet, my history of recurrent courses of antibiotics, living in a moldy apartment, and exposure to heavy metals were all contributing to my symptoms. In a quest to heal myself and to look for a better way to treat patients, I read and studied everything I could find related to these concepts. As I started to see more of my own patients in my residency training, I realized that quite a few of them were likely suffering from the same sorts of root causes as I was. I was no longer satisfied to hand out a prescription for each different symptom that they described. My goals for patients changed from making symptoms tolerable with medication to figuring out the cause of symptoms so they could be addressed, resulting in an automatic improvement in symptoms and overall well-being. I have seen how making lifestyle changes and discovering the causes of symptoms can result in significant improvement in the long-run. I have learned the importance of treating my mind/body/spirit with care, including the food I eat, the environment and people that I surround myself with and the thoughts that go through my mind. While staying balanced and healthy in our world today is quite a challenge, setting the intention to make this a priority is crucial to all of us.

As part of my ongoing educational journey, I had the good fortune of attending a seminar with Michael Lebowitz DC about 2 years ago. Subsequently, I had the opportunity to observe his practice for the past year and see how the techniques he has developed over the past 20 years can result in significant improvement in, if not complete remission from, symptoms ranging anywhere from an infant with colic, to a teenager suffering from Crohn's disease to an adult suffering from fibromyalgia. I was able to see first hand that natural therapies combined with lifestyle changes can result in improved health and quality of life for numerous patients.

My intent for this book is for it to serve as an educational tool for those who are suffering from some sort of ailment, as well as for those who are healthy, in an effort to educate patients about the causes of illness and what can be done to correct/avoid them. The second half of the book could also be viewed as an introductory lesson in functional medicine concepts for the practitioner who is curious to find a better way to address his/her patients' concerns.

I would like to thank Dr. Lebowitz for sharing his knowledge with me and for helping me improve my own health with his techniques; I hope to be able to offer patients' hope for recovery and help them overcome health challenges as he is able to do on a daily basis in his practice. I would like to thank Cynthia Lebowitz for her kindness and encouragement, as well as her numerous creations of healthy, allergy-friendly eating options that should soon be available in the Body Restoration Cookbook. I would also like to thank my parents, my brother Sheil, my sister Seema, my brother-in-law Justin and my friend Lydia who have always been there for me and encouraged me to pursue what has become my passion in holistic medicine.

Finally, I would like to offer hope to those who have lost it, and let them know that, regardless of your "diagnosis," it is possible for your body to restore itself with effort, time and perseverance.

Wishing you good health and happiness,

Ami Kapadia MD

PART 1:   ORGANS AND GLANDS

Chapter 1:   **ADRENAL GLANDS**

Anatomy and Physiology

The adrenals are two small glands, one on top of each kidney, with a total weight of about 1/3 of an ounce. Each has an outer layer called the medulla, which is related to our sympathetic nervous system. The medulla secretes epinephrine and norepinephrine (commonly known as adrenaline). The adrenals also each have an inner layer called the cortex, which secretes three different classes of hormones: mineralocorticoids, glucocorticoids, and androgenic hormones.

Anatomy and Physiology of the Adrenal Medulla

Many nerves from the sympathetic nervous system go to the adrenal medulla, and end on special cells that secrete epinephrine and norepinephrine whenever stimulated by these nerves. These hormones then travel through our circulatory system to all parts of our body. Some of the most important functions of epinephrine and norepinephrine include:

1) Speeding up the rate of metabolism of cells as much as 100%
2) Increasing blood pressure
3) Dilating the blood vessels to the heart and skeletal muscles, while constricting most other vessels
4) Increasing blood flow to the muscles while decreasing blood flow to organs not in use at the time
5) Causing the liver to release glucose, thus increasing blood glucose levels
6) Decreasing urine output
7) Dilating pupils
8) Increasing muscle strength and mental activity (partially due to increased glucose levels)
9) Dilation of bronchial pathways (this is why epinephrine injections are given during asthmatic attacks)
10) Breaking down glucose in muscles

Anatomy and Physiology of the Adrenal Cortex

Of the three different classes of hormones secreted by the adrenal cortex, aldosterone is the main mineralocorticoid, cortisol is the main glucocorticoid, and DHEA is the main androgenic hormone. We will focus mostly on aldosterone and cortisol, and briefly discuss DHEA/androgenic hormones.

Mineralocorticoid/Aldosterone:

Aldosterone is the chief mineralocorticoid. Aldosterone causes sodium retention and potassium excretion by the kidneys. If we had no aldosterone, we would die within two weeks. Our sodium and chloride ions would decrease, and the potassium level in the fluid surrounding our cells would increase. The lack of sodium and chloride would lead to decreased fluid and blood volume and eventually we would go into shock. The increased potassium level would also poison the heart.

On the other hand, too much aldosterone leads to increased sodium levels in the extra cellular fluids, as well as increased potassium excretion. Over long periods of time, this sodium/potassium imbalance would cause high blood pressure and muscle weakness. It would also cause the body to become overly alkaline.

Glucocorticoids/Cortisol:

The major glucocorticoids are cortisol (also known as hydrocortisone), corticosterone and cortisone. Most adrenocortical hormones are synthesized from cholesterol; therefore, when these hormones are called for by the body, cholesterol must be formed by the liver. This is one reason why stress increases serum cholesterol levels. Since all of the glucocorticoids have similar effects on the system, we will limit our discussion to cortisol (the major glucocorticoid).

Cortisol's main functions include the following:

1) Gluconeogenesis (Don't let long words scare you. Gluco means glucose, neo - new, genesis - beginning). Thus, cortisol is responsible for the body breaking down proteins and transporting amino acids

4

(the building blocks of protein) to the liver where they will be converted into "new sugar" or glucose. This is one way that cortisol contributes to elevated blood sugar levels.

2) Cortisol decreases the rate that cells use glucose, and decreases the rate glucose is brought to the cells. This is another way that cortisol contributes to elevated blood sugar levels, as it keeps glucose in your bloodstream rather than facilitating removal of glucose from the bloodstream and into the cells.

3) By the above mechanisms, cortisol increases blood glucose levels. Therefore, chronic excessive cortisol production or intake (cortisone pills and injections) can lead to a type of adrenal induced diabetes because of the chronically elevated blood sugar levels.

4) Excessive cortisol can depress the function of your immune system by shrinking thymus and lymph tissues and decreasing the activity and formation of lymphocytes, including natural killer cells, which are necessary to fight disease.

Adrenal hormone secretion is under control of the pituitary gland (see the pituitary chapter for more details). Almost any type of stress to the body will cause the anterior pituitary to signal the adrenals (via ACTH) to produce more cortisol. These can include:

1) Moderate to severe physical pain
2) Exposure to foods and other substances you are sensitive to
3) Dysbiosis (See the chapter on dysbiosis.)
4) Traumatic accidents (auto accidents, on the job injuries, etc.)
5) Taking epinephrine or norepinephrine (these are sometimes added to the anesthetic you get during your visit to the dentist)
6) Intense anxiety or emotional trauma (problems at work or home, divorce, death in family, etc.)
7) Overwork - mental or physical
8) Lack of proper sleep
9) Chronic diseases that wear down the body
10) Pollutants in our air, water, cleansers, deodorants, hair sprays, etc.
11) Pesticide and herbicide exposure
12) Refined foods, especially carbohydrates
13) Surgery
14) Extremes in temperature

Androgenic Hormones/DHEA:

The adrenals also produce male and female sex hormones in small amounts and these can influence your secondary sex characteristics, severity of menstruation, etc. The estrogen and progesterone are very important in women approaching menopause. If the adrenals are functioning properly, there is evidence that the body will slightly step up production of these hormones (or the hormone precursors) at menopause. This will slowly transition the body and make menopause fairly symptom free. In the multitudes of women that suffer from varying degrees of functional hypoadrenia (low adrenal function), menopause will be more severe with hot flashes, sweats, etc. (See the chapter on the ovaries for more information on menopause.)

The most abundant androgenic hormone produced by the adrenal cortex is DHEA or dehydroepiandrosterone. DHEA serves as a precursor to the male and female sex hormones, testosterone and estrogen, in appropriate tissues. DHEA helps to protect and increase bone density, keeps cholesterol levels in balance, provides energy and mental sharpness, and helps maintain normal sleep cycles. DHEA also helps the ability to recover from stress (emotional or physical). DHEA levels have been shown to decrease after the age of 30, and can be depleted by certain medications such as insulin, steroids, and opiates, among others. Decreased DHEA levels may also be seen in thyroid disorders, cardiovascular disease, obesity, reduced immunity, rheumatologic diseases, and with excess cortisol production. Low levels of DHEA are associated with a lowered capacity to endure physiological or psychological stress/trauma/injury. When DHEA levels are low, fatigue, irritability, dysglycemia, central obesity, impaired immunity, insomnia, depression, fatigue, decreased libido and osteoporosis may ensue.

Symptoms of Adrenal Malfunction

Due to our modern society, which has many physical and emotional stresses, probably over half the population possesses varying degrees of adrenal malfunction. As we are under stress for long periods of time, our adrenals produce extra cortisol and norepinephrine. Over time, our adrenals, by producing more hormones than they were made to comfortably manufacture and secrete, will "burn out" and decrease their secretion of these hormones. At that time of adrenal "burn out," the body loses its capacity to cope with stress; you become sick more easily and for longer periods of time, and perhaps even a nervous breakdown could result.

General symptoms of adrenal malfunction can include low back, sacroiliac, and knee pain, and tired feet with weak ankles and aching calves (you will probably exhibit a few but not all of the symptoms). Sprains and strains become more common. You will probably wear out the heels of your shoes more on the outside. Your eyes will be very sensitive to light, especially when driving at night, and you might feel a need to wear sunglasses during most summer days. Depression, hay fever, asthma, bronchitis, colitis, insomnia, learning disabilities, and ulcers (due to increased hydrochloric acid production) may all be partially due to adrenal malfunction. It is not uncommon for people with low adrenal function to feel dizzy when getting up quickly from a lying position.

If the major malfunction is with excessive production of aldosterone/mineralocorticoids, muscle spasms and possibly even convulsions could occur as well as systemic alkalosis (which would manifest in extreme nervousness). You might crave foods high in potassium.

Symptoms of a deficiency in aldosterone secretion (with resultant sodium loss) would include dehydration, excessive perspiration and urination, increased skin pigmentation, muscle twitching, and heart palpitations.

Excessive cortisol production due to prolonged stresses can decrease your immunity, leading to frequent and prolonged illnesses.

People that have a diminished output of cortisol can exhibit any of the following symptoms. They will crave substances that will temporarily raise their serum glucose level such as caffeine, sweets, soda or juice, tobacco, or marijuana. They may experience dizziness or brain fog. Irritability, headaches, blurred vision, erratic behavior and fluctuating energy levels may result. Since cortisol is an anti-inflammatory hormone, a decreased output over extended periods of time will make you prone to inflammatory diseases such as arthritis, bursitis, bronchitis, colitis, and allergies (many food and pollen allergies disappear when adrenal function is restored to normal). You will also have no reserve energy and infections can spread quickly.

A female suffering from increased output of androgens may develop excessive body hair and/or a deep voice. Cortisone derivatives are often given due to their function of suppression of adrenal function to treat this, but the side effects make it a treatment to avoid, if possible. In males, excessive androgens can lead to development of enlarged breasts.

Diminished epinephrine output can lead to bronchial restriction resulting in asthma, and can also alter thyroid function.

Hans Selye, often regarded as the father of modern stress/adrenal physiology, did an interesting experiment and showed that rats who had their adrenal glands removed were very prone to arthritis, but when they were given cortisol there were almost no instances of the disease (due to the side effects of taking cortisol injections, the ideal answer is to get your adrenals to produce a sufficient amount instead of relying on medications).

In my practice I have also seen that people with weak adrenals are more prone to ligamentous sprains when under physical stress than people with normal adrenals. Thus, it is especially important for athletes to keep their adrenals strong. This was first observed by Dr. George Goodheart, the founder of Applied Kinesiology.

Adrenal Malfunction

Hans Selye found that if you are under chronic, prolonged stress, your adrenal glands will go through a series of three stages. First, they will begin hyper-functioning to increase their hormone production and help you cope with the stress. With chronic stress, the glands will become overtaxed and depleted. If you are still fairly healthy at this point, the adrenals will rebuild themselves and actually hypertrophy (grow larger). But, if the stress continues (remember stress can be physical, emotional, thermal, environmental, nutritional, electromagnetic, etc.), the glands will again exhaust themselves and their functional capacity will decrease. At this point in time, you have no reserve capacity to handle stressful situations without overreacting or "going to pieces". It is our observation that in the process of rebuilding under-functioning glands (adrenals and most other endocrine glands), they will go through a period of hyper or over-functioning to try to catch up for lost time before returning to normal function.

Specific causes of adrenal malfunction:

1) Frequent ingestion of white sugar, honey, maple syrup, fruit juices, sodas, etc. will cause a rapid rise in blood glucose levels. Our bodies are not made to handle large amounts of concentrated sweets (an ice cream sundae has 24 teaspoons of sugar) and this rapid rise will cause the pancreas to "freak out" and overreact in insulin secretion - leading to a rapid fall in blood glucose levels. At that point, the adrenals must put out large amounts of cortisol to bring the blood sugar back to normal. This type of diet, which is very prevalent today, will over time exhaust the adrenals and also lead to hypoglycemia.

   One of the adrenal glucocorticoids (11-hydroxycorticosterone) is temporarily increased up to 400% by excessive white sugar ingestion. To restate, this can lead to both adrenal exhaustion and immune system depression.

2) Caffeine, alcohol and marijuana will have the same effect as the concentrated sweets listed above.

3) Eating foods you are sensitive to can stress the adrenals and lead to dysfunction. (See the chapter on food allergies/toxins.) Many people feel that eating too many trans/hydrogenated fats can impair adrenal function. These include margarine, hardened vegetable oils, etc.

4) The adrenals can also be overtaxed by sudden or prolonged exposure to heat or cold, not enough sleep, mental trauma, chronic disease and/or exposure to toxins and pollutants.

5) Infections, such as parasitic, viral, fungal, spirochete and bacterial infections can also stress the adrenal glands and lead to dysfunction. (See the chapter on dysbiosis.)

6) Taking cortisone in injection form is common in inflammatory conditions of the joints and hydrocortisone creams for itching and rashes are sold over the counter. In addition, oral steroid hormones are given in the form of prednisone for inflammatory conditions such as chronic obstructive pulmonary disease (COPD) and rheumatoid arthritis. Taking cortisone in these forms over prolonged periods of time could depress adrenal function and even lead to adrenal atrophy. Taking supplemental forms of cortisone can inhibit the production of corticotrophin releasing factor from the hypothalamus and ACTH production from the anterior pituitary. This in turn decreases cortisol production by the adrenal cortex. Inhaled steroids

given for asthma, etc. can possibly have similar effects. These drugs can be life saving at times, but can also be overprescribed. Treating dysbiosis, food sensitivities and adrenal malfunction naturally will bring optimal results that are long lasting and without side effects.

While occasional medication use is unlikely to be harmful, chronic use of cortisone type medication can have many adverse side effects in addition to and as a result of the adrenal suppression described above. Possible adverse reactions to chronic steroid use include: steroid psychosis, hypertension, loss of muscle mass, osteoporosis, peptic ulcer (steroids cause an increase in hydrochloric acid production by the stomach), impaired wound healing, convulsions, dizziness, headaches, diabetes, cataracts, glaucoma, weakened ligaments, etc.

The ideal way to approach the problem is to strengthen your own adrenal glands so they secrete enough cortisol and epinephrine to handle emergencies and prevent most problems (listed in symptom section as caused by weak adrenals).

7) Spinal misalignment in the lower thoracic spine and elsewhere may decrease adrenal function.
8) A problem with pituitary function can alter ACTH production and affect adrenal function. (See the chapter on the pituitary.)
9) Positively charged air from most heating and air conditioning systems can possibly depress adrenal function. Studies on hamsters showed that excessive exposure to positive ions decreased the weight of their adrenal glands.
10) The stress of pregnancy can aggravate a case of hypoadrenia. This can cause problems in the fetus. It is hypothesized that in the third trimester when the fetus starts producing its own adrenal hormones, a mother suffering from hypoadrenia, not having enough of her own adrenal hormones, will "rob" hormones from the fetus. The mother, as a result, will feel better until after she gives birth and she loses the extra hormone supply. Meanwhile, the fetus' adrenals, being forced to produce enough hormones for it and an adult, will get quickly depleted. The excess hormone production will also depress the baby's immune system. The infant will become very prone to allergies and recurrent infections, and be very irritable. The mother will often suffer from post partum depression when she no longer has access to

the baby's hormones.

11) A study done by Dr. William Raab showed that norepinephrine and epinephrine production would rise dramatically while watching exciting television shows. The side effects, including higher blood pressure, would last for several hours. A "diet" of lots of these shows could exhaust the adrenal medulla and under real stress, when you need these hormones in large amounts, they might not be available. This could possibly also hold true for certain video games and other activities.

12) If your adrenals are already somewhat depleted, going on a fast can sometimes worsen the condition. The adrenals must stay very active during a fast to maintain your blood glucose level and they could get further overtaxed. With low adrenal function, healthy snacks like raw nuts, or whole fresh fruits and vegetables can help stabilize blood sugar in between meals without overtaxing the adrenals.

Other Indications of Adrenal Malfunction

1) With normal epinephrine secretion, when you shine a light into your pupil, the pupil should constrict for at least thirty seconds. In cases of decreased secretion it will dilate, alternately open and close, or constrict for less than thirty seconds.

2) Normal tongues should feel slick. If aldosterone is low your tongue may have another feeling.

3) Normally, when you rise quickly from a prone position, norepinephrine and cortisol are secreted. This causes constriction of abdominal blood vessels and a resultant rise in blood pressure of about 1-5mm Hg. In people with hypoadrenia, the blood pressure will drop, even up to 20 points, and dizziness will occur. To do this test, have the patient lie down and relax for 4-5 minutes. Take their blood pressure and leave the cuff on (deflated), then have them rise quickly and retake it as soon as possible. You can use this as a monitoring device if you are treating your adrenals to see if you are improving.

Prevention and Correction of Adrenal Malfunction

Symptoms of adrenal malfunction can start improving as soon as 2-3 days after commencement of therapy or it could be 2-3 months before any improvement is seen in resistant cases. The harder cases are people who have been on cortisone, epinephrine, or allergy medication, along with alcoholics, sugarholics, people addicted to caffeine, marijuana, etc. Also, if you do not identify and treat dysbiosis and food sensitivities it will be much harder and sometimes impossible to correct adrenal function. With patience, I've seen wonderful results in even the most difficult cases. Remember, if instructions (especially dietary restrictions) are not closely adhered to, progress can be slow or nil. A food binge midway through the program can slow progress greatly and cause the need for much additional therapy to start the healing process again.

1) One of the most important steps in either preventing malfunction or regenerating tired adrenals is what I call the adrenal recovery diet. For 1-2 months the following foods must be eliminated - sugar (white, brown, and "raw"), honey, molasses, corn syrup, maple syrup, etc., also dried fruit and fruit juices. No alcohol, drugs, tobacco, or caffeine, are allowed. Trans fats should be avoided. Fresh fruit is allowed. After 1-2 months, if you feel significant improvement, small amounts of honey, molasses, dried fruit, and fruit juice, are allowed. But until then, 100% compliance is very important. If you buy prepared food read the labels carefully; if it has sweetening, don't get it (stevia is allowed). Breads can be made using unsweetened applesauce or cooked sweet potato to make the yeast rise. Many of the more rustic breads (French, batards, bouls, ciabatta, etc), pocket breads, chapattis, Essene bread, etc. don't use any sweetening but you will need to read labels. Again, the stricter you are, the better and faster your results will be. During the first one or two weeks on this diet some people (usually the more severe cases) go through what I call withdrawal. Symptoms can include irritability, feeling edgy, craving sweets and feeling like you're going crazy. If this happens, please grin and bear it, it will eventually pass and then you will improve rapidly. Your body is doing without the chemicals and refined products it is addicted to, and in the beginning it is a hard transition. With patience and determination, you will be successful.

2) Try to trace the problem down to its cause (see the section on causes) and eliminate it if at all possible.

3) Get enough sleep. Going to bed by 9-10PM is ideal, as is having at least 8 hours of sleep.

4) It is necessary to figure out and eliminate all food allergies/food toxins. (See the chapter on food allergies/food toxins.)

5) It is necessary to find and treat all chronic, subclinical infections. (See the chapter on chronic infections.)

6) Don't fast. Eat healthy between meal snacks like raw nuts or vegetables.

7) Stay off medications containing cortisone and epinephrine if possible. If you are on them, consult with a holistically oriented physician to see if it is possible to wean yourself off (do not do this on your own, only do it under medical supervision).

8) Stand in the shower with your back facing the spray and have it beat down on your adrenals (just above the kidneys). Do 3 minutes of the hottest water you can stand followed by 30 seconds of the coldest, once daily.

9) Cup your hand and tap hard on the skin overlapping the adrenal glands for 2 minutes daily.

10) Evaluate the need for treating the pituitary, thyroid, liver, and pancreas, as one or more could also be involved and need treating simultaneously or later on in the future. For example, if the adrenals are malfunctioning secondary to pituitary malfunction, it is the pituitary that needs work. Or, if you're not making enough cortisol it will tax the glucagon production of the pancreas to keep your blood sugar up, and the pancreas may eventually need work too. (See their respective chapters.)

11) Have a good chiropractor check for spinal misalignment and correct it (I personally prefer one knowledgeable in Applied Kinesiology, though there are also many other fine techniques that can do the job).

12) Vigorously rub a reflex point (called a neuro-lymphatic reflex) located 2 inches above and 1 inch to each side of the umbilicus for 1 minute 3 times a week. They will probably be tender if the adrenals are malfunctioning.

13) During stressful times, lie down and relax and place your hands on your forehead over your eyebrows. Stay like that for 10 minutes. It will be very calming.

14) Get out in the fresh air and let new air circulate in your house. Air charged with negative ions is healing to the adrenals. This air is abundant in the forest, seashore and mountains.

15) Get out in the sunshine. The latest research suggests that sunlight striking the skin produces small amounts of epinephrine. This could help an overworked adrenal.

16) The proper amount of melatonin secretion by the pineal gland may aid the adrenals in combating stress. Getting to bed early is helpful for optimum production. (See the chapter on the pineal gland.)

17) Decrease your stress.

18) Minimize exposure to toxins and pollutants.
19) Dress properly for warmth and health. Clothe your extremities if it's not very hot out.

I'd like to briefly discuss 3 cases of adrenal malfunction I have seen over the years to give you an idea of the symptoms, results, etc.

A 4-year-old girl was brought in by her parents because once or twice daily she would throw an awful temper tantrum. It had been going on for about a year and the parents had no patience left to deal with it. After taking a careful history and doing a thorough exam, it appeared she was suffering from hypoadrenia and a food sensitivity to soy products. We treated the reflex points listed in this section, put her on the adrenal recovery diet, and had her eliminate all forms of soy. They came back one month later and reported that for the whole month she had only one tantrum and that she seemed like a totally different girl. After testing, it seemed her stronger adrenals had relieved her food sensitivity to soy (sometimes, though not always, food allergies are secondary and by correcting dysbiosis, nutrient deficiencies and organ dysfunction, the food reactions can be eliminated). We put her back on soy and allowed small quantities of juice, dried fruit, and honey back into the diet. The honey was used mainly in cooking where it was only a minor ingredient. She was able to handle it as long as her intake wasn't excessive. About two months later she had a lot of sugary cookies at a neighbor's house and threw two tantrums. We reworked the reflexes and she was fine again. Since then, the tantrums haven't returned and her adrenals are strong enough now to handle occasional dietary divergences on special occasions.

Another patient had an intolerance to gluten (in wheat, rye, etc.) so much so that just a bite or two would keep him miserably congested for weeks and he would feel like he was "on drugs", with severe brain fog. All the doctors that he saw agreed that he'd have to abstain from gluten for the rest of his life. Again, after determining hypoadrenia to be a major factor we put him on the adrenal recovery diet, used the reflex points, hot and cold showers, and adrenal tapping. After 2 weeks he seemed to be much stronger and he went ahead and had bread and a bowl of noodles with no reaction and has been fine since. In many cases these food intolerances are life long but in this case the gluten intolerance was secondary.

I was one of my toughest cases. On allergy shots weekly for many years, daily antihistamines, and a diet with unlimited cakes, pies, and ice cream, my adrenals were exhausted. My capacity to handle stress was nonexistent. I was irritable, very depressed, tired, had many headaches, excessive urination, and craved sweets frequently, along with having erratic behavior. I gave up the shots and medication in 1970, but eating wheat, corn, dairy, or potatoes would congest me terribly as would exposure to pollen. I could easily saturate a dozen handkerchiefs daily and often had to sleep with one stuffed up my nose. After 4 months on the diet, and using the reflex points, most of my symptoms were gone, though I still had the headaches and occasional congestion. Today I'd say the symptoms are 97% gone. I don't follow the adrenal recovery diet as strictly anymore. I occasionally have dried fruit or honey, maple syrup etc., yet keep them to a minimum. I notice that if I do not follow it for 3-4 days in a row - I can develop a food sensitivity and get congested. I also had to treat a chronic subclinical fungal infection (see the chapter on dysbiosis) and correct a mold situation in our house to help stabilize things.

Once you have had severe hypoadrenia you always have to be careful with your diet, exercise, etc. You can never go back to a junk food diet without suffering, but you learn to relish the taste of natural foods. The old cravings leave and the restoration of health and happiness is well worth it. Again, get enough sleep, as this step is too often neglected.

Supplement Recommendations - in chapters when we list supplements we are not suggesting you take them all. Usually only one or two are indicated. Have your natural health care practitioner help with your decision or, if you do not have one, do some trials on your own.

THORNE RESEARCH

    1) L-Tyrosine

    2) Cortrex

    3) B Complex #5

    4) Phytisone

SUPREME NUTRITION PRODUCTS

5) Endo Supreme

6) Camu Supreme

7) Reishi Supreme

8) Ashwaganda Supreme (unless you are solanine sensitive, in which case you should avoid Ashwaganda as it is a solanine) (See the food toxin and supplements chapters.)

9) Additional supplements will most likely be needed to correct dysbiosis. (See the dysbiosis chapter.)

I cannot stress enough that subclinical infections and food sensitivities/intolerances must be addressed to get long lasting resolution to most adrenal problems. (See their respective chapters.)

Chapter 2:   **THYROID GLAND**

Anatomy and Physiology

The thyroid gland is located just below the larynx and in front of and to the side of the trachea.

Thyroid hormones act on virtually every cell in the body. We will be discussing three major hormones secreted by the thyroid. The first two, thyroxine (T4) and triiodothyronine (T3), are primarily controlled by thyroid stimulating hormone (TSH) secreted by the anterior pituitary gland. TSH production, in turn, is modulated by thyrotropin releasing hormone (TRH) secretion from the hypothalamus. The third hormone released from the thyroid gland, calcitonin, is not under hypothalamic/pituitary control. Calcitonin is involved in calcium homeostasis and responds to calcium levels in the blood.

Of the thyroid hormones released from the thyroid gland, about 80% are in the form of T4 and 20% in the form of T3. Up to 80% of the T4 released from the thyroid gland is converted to the more active T3 by peripheral organs such as the liver and kidney. T3 is a more potent hormone (approximately four times as strong), but T4 is much longer lasting. At any given time, most of the T4 and T3 in the body are bound to transport proteins; it is only the small, "unbound" or "free" portion of the hormones that is biologically active.

The thyroid gland needs about 1/5000th of a gram of iodine daily to be used in the formation of these two hormones. Tyrosine is also required to make thyroid hormones.

The functions of thyroxine and triiodothyronine are as follows:

1) Increase the basal metabolic rate of the body, thus setting the rate of the chemical reactions that occur in the body
2) Increase the rate at which the body uses food for energy, thus playing an important role in determining your caloric requirement
3) Increase the rate at which the body both makes and breaks down

glucose (gluconeogenesis and glycolysis), thus increasing the absorption of glucose by the cells in general and by the gastrointestinal tract

4) Increase insulin secretion by the pancreas
5) Increase the respiration rate and depth of each breath
6) Increase the rate of both protein synthesis and breakdown
7) Increase the growth rate of adolescents while quickening the closing rate of epiphyses in bones
8) Increase fat deposition into circulation to be burned for energy
9) Increase appetite
10) Increase urinary excretion of calcium and phosphorus
11) Increase secretion of digestive enzymes and peristalsis in the gastrointestinal tract
12) Dilate blood vessels, thus increasing blood flow
13) Increase heart rate, body temperature, and systolic blood pressure while decreasing diastolic pressure

The parafollicular cells of the thyroid gland secrete the third thyroid hormone, calcitonin.

When levels of calcium in the blood are too high, calcitonin is secreted and has the following effects:

1) Stimulates the movement of calcium into bone (in opposition to the effects of parathyroid hormone)
2) Increases the activity of bone forming cells (osteoblasts)
3) Decreases the activity and formation of cells that break down bone (osteoclasts). This process helps build new bone and lower serum calcium, which in turn, stops calcitonin secretion.

Because of the close relationship between calcitonin and parathyroid hormone of the parathyroid gland, most of our discussion involving symptoms, causes, etc. of calcium disturbance will be in the chapter on the parathyroid gland.

Symptoms of Thyroid Dysfunction

A person secreting too little thyroxine and/or triiodothyronine can exhibit some of the following symptoms:

1) They will often be overweight and have a hard time losing weight, even with a restricted caloric intake, due to a decreased metabolic rate.

2) The decreased metabolic rate will also make them require more sleep and even when awake they will be tired and exhibit very little motivation and ambition. They will tend to have difficulty getting out of bed in the morning and can exhibit a poor memory.

3) They may tend to build up cholesterol deposits and be more prone to heart troubles. The sluggish circulation will also manifest in having cold hands and feet.

4) Too little thyroid hormone production can lead to an imbalanced output of estrogen and progesterone by the ovaries, leading to prolonged and painful periods, with an increased tendency towards water retention.

5) A decreased depth of respiration will make it easy for the person to get out of breath with just a little bit of exertion.

6) Decreased peristalsis may lead to constipation.

7) A person with hypothyroidism will get depressed easily and often cry or go to pieces from situations that do not warrant these reactions.

8) Other symptoms observed with this condition include: balding or thinning of hair, brittle nails, hands and feet that tend to peel or crack, chapped lips, decreased resistance to infections and a tendency to get muscle cramps easily.

9) Because sudden temperature or seasonal changes put the thyroid under stress in hypothyroid people, they will exhibit increased health problems at these times.

A person over-secreting thyroid hormones can exhibit some or all of the following:

1) They will have trouble putting on weight (they will often be quite thin and wiry).

2) They will be nervous, worry a lot and have a hard time falling asleep (even when tired).

3) They will tend to sweat most of the time and dislike the heat.

4) They will have a tendency toward diarrhea (see the chapter on the large intestine for other causes of diarrhea).

5) More severe cases may possibly exhibit hand tremors and protrusion of the eyeballs.

Causes of Thyroid Dysfunction

1) It is the author's clinical experience that hypothyroidism is often due to a deficiency of the amino acid tyrosine which converts into T3 and T4. For some reason, we find many more women need tyrosine than men. It is depleted by stress and is not assimilated well in the diet unless starch and protein meals are separated. L-tyrosine supplementation will usually correct hormone levels and prescription hormones can often be avoided. This is typically only true if it is tried before prescription hormones are taken or if the person has only been on them a few months.

2) Chronic subclinical infections, such as parasitic, viral, fungal, spirochete and bacterial infections can also stress the thyroid gland and lead to dysfunction. (See the chapter on dysbiosis.)

3) Eating foods you are allergic to can stress the thyroid gland and lead to dysfunction. (See the chapter on food allergies/food toxins.)

4) It is the author's observation that toxic metal exposure, especially mercury, can lead to abnormal thyroid function. (See the chapter on heavy metals.)

5) Because of the thyroid's effect on insulin secretion, prolonged intake of refined carbohydrates and sweets can cause the overtaxing of your thyroid gland and lead to dysfunction. Our bodies were not designed to handle large amounts of refined products and physiologically we pay the consequences when overindulging.

6) Because of the resultant change in endocrine output with prolonged use, taking birth control pills, epinephrine and/or cortisone can lead to thyroid dysfunction.

7) Taking synthetic thyroid hormone for an inactive thyroid gland will tend to make your thyroid rely more on this outside source and will thus lead to further inactivity. It makes so much more sense to us to look for and correct the cause of the dysfunction in an effort to allow the thyroid to heal and return to normal functioning.

8) Overeating, especially fats and sugars, over prolonged periods will make the body produce more thyroid hormones (to increase fat burning and glucose uptake) than it can comfortably produce. This can eventually lead to hypothyroidism.

9) X-rays striking the thyroid (including dental x-rays) can damage the thyroid.

10) Prolonged, excessive intake of vitamin A supplements and also zinc can lead to hypothyroidism.

11) A lack of iodine in the diet can lead to dysfunction.

12) An imbalance in the amount of estrogen in the body (be it due to pituitary, liver, ovary, or adrenal malfunction) can alter thyroid function.

13) Excess intake of cruciferous vegetables can lower thyroid function in some people.

14) If you suffer from hypoadrenia (see the adrenal chapter), the thyroid will often slow down to decrease your metabolic rate and give the adrenals a chance to rest.

15) Spinal misalignment in the mid cervical spine can cause thyroid dysfunction. I have seen it time after time in patients of mine involved in car accidents with resultant whiplash and cervical nerve dysfunction: they will go into a state of hypothyroidism and put on 10-30 pounds over the next 3-4 months.

16) Various strong emotional states can affect TSH secretion and cause thyroid hormone output to change. If this emotional state isn't properly dealt with, thyroid dysfunction will eventually result. Other causes of pituitary dysfunction can cause thyroid disturbances secondary to pituitary malfunction. (See the pituitary chapter.) In these cases, the pituitary must be restored to normal function in order for the thyroid to also be restored.

17) Increased exposure to the cold, especially without properly clothing the extremities, will (via the hypothalamus and pituitary) cause an increase in thyroid hormone output, which over time can overwork the thyroid and lead to dysfunction.

Other Indications of Thyroid Dysfunction

Not all cases of thyroid dysfunction will show up on blood tests. An easy way to check your metabolic rate at home and get a general idea of your thyroid function involves keeping a temperature chart. Every morning, before you get out of bed, take your axillary temperature. Put the bulb of the thermometer in your armpit and with your arm tightly against your body keep it there for a full five minutes. Record the temperature daily for one month and find the average. A normal axillary temperature would be between 97.6-98.4. If it is less and you exhibit some of the symptoms mentioned in the hypothyroid section, you could have an under-functioning gland. If over 98.4 and symptoms match, you could have an over-functioning thyroid. There are many other causes of altered body temperature so do not rely on this as a sole diagnosis.

Treatment of Thyroid Dysfunction

If your thyroid has been surgically removed, you will need to take medication. If it hasn't been removed, it is the author's opinion that medication should only be taken if all else fails, as it may further inhibit the body's own production of thyroid hormones and might possibly produce side effects. First off, try to prevent the thyroid from dysfunctioning, but if it is too late, try to help the thyroid heal and restore its normal function.

1) It is necessary to figure out and eliminate all food allergies/food toxins. (See the chapter on food allergies/food toxins.)
2) It is necessary to find and treat all chronic, subclinical infections. (See the chapter on dysbiosis.)
3) It is necessary to figure out if there is a component of heavy metal toxicity and address it. (See the chapter on heavy metals.)
4) Abstain from alcohol, caffeine, marijuana, tobacco, birth control pills, and other drugs that may harm the thyroid. (Consult your physician before stopping any prescription medications.)
5) Minimize intake of white sugar, brown sugar, molasses, corn syrup, margarine, vegetable oil, and other refined sugars and hydrogenated fats. Don't overeat.
6) If you must be x-rayed, make sure the thyroid is properly shielded.
7) When it is cold, make sure your whole body is dressed warmly.
8) Decrease the stress in your life.
9) If you've had a whiplash injury or suspect spinal misalignment, have a good chiropractor check it out.
10) Make sure your pituitary, adrenals, pancreas, reproductive glands, and liver are functioning properly and not causing secondary thyroid disturbances.
11) Since most soils are somewhat depleted, if you have a garden, consider fertilizing with liquid seaweed or fish emulsion to supply iodine to the soil. Care must be exhibited as these can sometimes be a source of mercury.
12) There are 2 reflex points that may help normalize thyroid function, one on each side of the sternum (breastbone) between the 2nd and 3rd ribs. Rub them vigorously for one to two minutes, two times weekly, for one month.
13) A treatment that may help thyroid function is to take a very hot compress and put it over the thyroid for 30 seconds and then put an

ice bag there for 30 seconds. Alternate hot and ice 6 times, once in the morning and once at night, for one week.

14) For an under-functioning thyroid, you should stay away from excessive vitamin A (more than 10,000 IU vitamin A daily) and excessive zinc (more than 30 mg zinc daily) supplementation. Decrease foods with thiourea (thyroid inhibitor) - these include cabbage, broccoli, cauliflower, kohlrabi, peanuts and soybeans. Eat food high in iodine and manganese (seaweed, seeds, dark green vegetables, kale, collards, etc.). Some people do not tolerate iodine well, so be careful. Oats and bananas can be helpful because they stimulate the thyroid. A cold short bath, or a sunbath, and lots of vigorous physical exercise will all help revive a sluggish thyroid.

15) For an over functioning thyroid gland, an ice bag for 30 minutes daily will help slow it down temporarily. Eat foods high in thiourea - cabbage, broccoli, cauliflower, kohlrabi, soybeans, and peanuts. Avoid bananas and oats.

16) For an under-functioning thyroid , try taking an L-Tyrosine supplement (500mg. on rising and 500mg. mid morning) and a natural iodine supplement like Alaria Supreme.

Supplement Recommendations

THORNE RESEARCH

    1) Tyrosine

    2) Iodine-Tyrosine

    3) Thyroscin

SUPREME NUTRITION PRODUCTS

    4) Endo Supreme

    5) Alaria Supreme

Michael Lebowitz DC and Ami Kapadia MD

Chapter 3: **PANCREAS** (INSULIN AND GLUCAGON)

Anatomy and Physiology

The pancreas is composed of two major types of tissue. The acinar cells secrete digestive enzymes and will be discussed in a later chapter. Our present concern is the Islets of Langerhans, which contain insulin producing beta cells and glucagon producing alpha cells. The pancreas is about 6 inches long and weighs approximately 3 ounces. It is located at the level of the first lumbar vertebra, and parts of it touch the aorta, left kidney, left adrenal, and spleen.

Insulin has the following functions:

1) It increases the rate of glucose metabolism. Glucose that is not needed immediately by the cells is changed into glycogen for storage (in the liver, skeletal muscles, and skin), and fat (especially for storage in the adipose tissue and liver). A condition called "insulin resistance" is on the rise. Insulin resistance is a condition where the body is still making insulin, but cannot use it properly. Muscle, fat and liver cells do not respond as they should to insulin. As a result, more than the usual amount of insulin is needed to help glucose enter cells. The pancreas ends up producing more insulin to try and keep up, but eventually the cells become so resistant that simply increasing the amount of insulin is no longer enough. Over time, insulin resistance can lead to type II diabetes.
2) It decreases the glucose level in the blood and increases glucose transport to skeletal muscle, heart, smooth muscle and fat cells. It does not affect glucose transport to the brain or red blood cells.
3) It increases transport of amino acids into the cells and causes an increase in protein synthesis.
4) It works along with growth hormone to promote growth.

With a lack of insulin, the liver will start breaking down glycogen and forming new glucose (gluconeogenesis). Fats will also be released into the blood in the form of free fatty acids. Amino acids will be released into the blood and very little protein synthesis will take place. Over time, with a lack of insulin, acetone and ketone bodies will occur (due to largely burning fats instead of carbohydrates). This can lead to a state of acidosis. Also "protein wasting" occurs and can lead to extreme weakness, weight loss and organ dysfunction.

If a diet high in sugar (especially refined sugars, molasses, maple syrup, too much honey, and fruit juice) is eaten, the blood glucose level increases rapidly. A diet consistently high in sugar and other refined sweets will first lead to hypertrophy of the beta cells (to increase insulin production) and eventual burnout, with diabetes being a possible result.

Glucagon is secreted by the alpha cells of the Islets of Langerhans. Its main function is to break down glycogen into glucose and to stimulate gluconeogenesis; thus, increasing the blood glucose level. When blood glucose levels drop below 70 mg per 100 ml of blood, glucagon is secreted in large quantities to prevent hypoglycemia and make sure the brain is getting enough glucose (its major nutrient). If left uncontrolled, glucagon could deplete the liver of glycogen within four hours. Epinephrine and cortisol released by the adrenals also raise blood sugar, as does growth hormone from the anterior pituitary.

We can see how the adrenals, pancreas, thyroid, pituitary, and liver are all critical in keeping our blood sugar levels stable, and often an abnormal condition resulting in a blood sugar handling problem is due to a malfunction in more than one organ or gland.

Symptoms of Pancreas Malfunction

General symptoms that may indicate pancreatic malfunction include:

1) Headaches
2) Cold extremities
3) Increased sweating
4) Pain on the whole left side of the body
5) Sluggishness

Symptoms of low blood sugar from excess insulin secretion or from too little glucagon, epinephrine or cortisol (thus there may be multiple organ involvement) can include: feeling faint, tired, restless, weak, irritable, shaky, depressed and light headed. The person will often awaken in the middle of the night and have trouble falling back asleep.

A person with low blood sugar tends to have a poor memory, craves sweets, may have a rapid heartbeat, be prone to asthma or allergies, have poor concentration and a hard time learning. This type of person usually feels better after eating.

Symptoms of high blood sugar from inadequate insulin secretion, insulin resistance or too much glucagon, cortisol, or epinephrine include: weakness, nausea, headaches, shortness of breath, increased thirst, acidosis, ketosis, increased urination and dehydration, diarrhea and mood swings. In cases of diabetes, there is glucose in the urine, an increased likelihood of eye diseases (in diabetes the retina, which is completely dependent on glucose for energy, doesn't get the amount it needs) including blindness, kidney disease, heart disease and peripheral nerve diseases. Insulin dependent diabetics have their life spans decreased by as many as thirty years.

Causes of Pancreas Malfunction

1) With very few exceptions - the foods God placed on the earth have much lower sugar concentrations than the foods man has invented. While a watermelon may be 5% sugar and a banana 20%, ketchup can be 30-50%, salad dressings and breakfast cereal up to 50% or more. These man made sweet foods tend to make the pancreas overreact and produce too much insulin. The resultant drop in blood sugar leads us to crave sweets, thus we grab a snack and the cycle repeats itself. In the beginning, the resultant hypertrophy of the beta cells leads to a hypoglycemic state, but after years of overindulgence, the beta cells burn out and diabetes can result. This type of diet also does damage to the adrenals, thyroid, liver, pituitary, immune system, etc. Too many sweets as well as trans fats, refined carbohydrates etc. can lead to insulin resistance.

2) Caffeine, chocolate, smoking, alcohol and marijuana will have similar effects to concentrated sweets.

3) Eating too often in between meals won't let the pancreas rest and can lead to its exhaustion. Three meals daily with little or nothing in between is ideal. Overeating has the same effects.

4) Oral contraceptives, thiazides (diuretics used often to treat high blood

pressure), corticosteroids (cortisone etc.), caffeine, nicotine and overdosing on niacin supplements all increase blood glucose levels and thus alter pancreatic secretions. Over time, this could cause pancreatic dysfunction. The following also alter glucose metabolism and over long periods of time could alter pancreatic function: sulfa drugs, alcohol, and oral ingestion of growth hormone.

5) Insulin injections are necessary in cases of Type I diabetes. Type II diabetes is sometimes controllable without insulin or other medications if the patient is willing to make lifestyle changes. If we take insulin injections, it gives our body less reason to produce our own insulin, and many feel the beta cells slowly atrophy. Before going on insulin for adult onset diabetes, it is our opinion that we should try to rejuvenate our pancreas so it produces enough insulin, and follow better lifestyle practices to ensure a healthy body and proper utilization of our insulin. Even in cases of juvenile onset diabetes, insulin doses can be kept down by a proper lifestyle. You should only do this in conjunction with your physician.

6) There is a hereditary component to diabetes. We usually inherit a *predisposition* toward diabetes, but proper diet, exercise, etc., can often stop the disease from developing even if the tendency is there. There are cases of identical twins where only one develops Type I diabetes. Some recent theories say that certain forms of dysbiosis, especially viral, may contribute to the onset of diabetes as can a dairy allergy or possibly other foods in susceptible individuals.

7) In many cases, what is thought to be hereditary may be related to a mother's lifestyle. A diabetic pregnant woman on a poor diet may increase the likelihood of her child developing the same condition if the genetics are already in place.

8) In studies of isolated tribes living on diets of only unrefined foods, diabetes is virtually nonexistent. In some of these societies, white sugar, white flour, etc. have been introduced and within a few years up to one third of the adult population has shown signs of diabetes.

9) Leucine is an amino acid found in large concentrations in dairy products. In some sensitive individuals, ingestion of high leucine foods can cause a substantial change in blood sugar. With continued use of dairy, the pancreas is overtaxed and altered function results. Very few total vegetarians are diabetic compared to lacto-ovo-vegetarians. Other research has shown that eating foods you are sensitive to can dramatically raise blood sugar in susceptible patients.

10) Exercise and sunlight both have positive effects in balancing blood

sugar. Lack of these can contribute to problems.

11) Spinal misalignment in the mid thoracics can lead to pancreas malfunction.

Treatment and Prevention of Pancreas Malfunction

1) In general, we have often seen normalization in blood sugar levels if dysbiosis is corrected and food sensitivities are avoided.

2) Follow the adrenal recovery diet listed in the adrenal chapter. Eat no dairy products. Don't use artificial sweeteners. Eat 3 meals daily spaced at least 5 hours apart, with only water or unsweetened herb tea between meals.

3) Try to reach and maintain your ideal weight.

4) In type II diabetes, a fast for 4-7 days followed by the before mentioned diet will often partially or totally bring down elevated blood sugar. This should be done only under a doctor's supervision.

5) Have a good chiropractor see if spinal misalignment is a contributory cause. And in general try to trace down the cause and eliminate it.

6) Occasionally, chromium supplements may help, especially in gestational diabetes.

7) A one minute hot compress followed by thirty seconds of ice, alternate four times. Do this twice daily over the pancreas and mid thoracic spine. This will tend to normalize pancreatic secretions while you search out the cause and correct your lifestyle.

8) Sunbaths will cause the body (if your blood sugar is high) to convert glucose to glycogen and thus lower your blood glucose level. Caution: diabetics on insulin may need less insulin if they get an abundance of sun exposure.

9) Exercise will decrease blood sugar in diabetics and raise it in hypoglycemics. At least 30-40 minutes of vigorous exercise 5-6 times a week is needed.

10) Short cold baths are beneficial to diabetics (extremely hot baths should be avoided).

11) Vigorously rub a point between the 7th and 8th ribs on the left where the ribs and cartilage meet for 1 minute daily every other day.

12) For diabetics, the following herb teas are reported as beneficial: mullein, uva ursi, and cedar berries. String bean juice is also good.

13) Get enough rest, drink 6-8 glasses of water daily, and get lots of fresh air.

Chapter 4: **PITUITARY GLAND**

Anatomy & Physiology

The pituitary gland is located at the base of the brain in a pocket inside the sphenoid bone known as the sella turcica. It weighs only 1/2 gram (.018 ounces) of which 85% is water and it produces 1/100,000th of a gram of hormones daily.

The pituitary gland via hormone secretion directly affects the thyroid, adrenals, ovaries, testes, kidneys and breasts. According to *An Endocrine Interpretation of Chapman's Reflexes*: the pituitary "also exerts a definite influence on the intestines, bladder, uterus, stomach, and spleen, its actions causing contraction of the plain, unstrained muscles of the entire body".

Pituitary secretions are for the most part in response to signals from the hypothalamus. The hypothalamus communicates with the posterior pituitary via nerve fibers and the anterior pituitary via minute capillaries. The hypothalamus collects information from the body concerning hormone and electrolyte levels, pain, emotions, etc. and signals the pituitary accordingly with the optimum health of the body in mind.

There are six major hormones secreted by the anterior pituitary: adrenocorticotropic hormone (ACTH), thyroid stimulating hormone (TSH), follicle stimulating hormone (FSH), luteinizing hormone (LH), growth hormone (GH), and prolactin.

ACTH stimulates cortisol secretion by the adrenal glands and can increase its secretion up to 2000%. It also has a small effect on aldosterone and perhaps estrogen secretion. ACTH can be stimulated by low blood sugar, infection, surgery, chronic disease, intense heat or cold, norepinephrine and similar medications.

TSH signals the thyroid to secrete thyroxine and triiodothyronine. It also increases the production of these hormones and increases the size and number of thyroid cells. Two factors that cause abnormally high TSH secretion are intense cold and emotional trauma.

FSH in males aids in formation of sperm and in females aids in the development of the egg and production of estrogen. (See the chapter on ovaries for more information.)

LH in males stimulates the formation of testosterone and in females it is necessary for follicular growth, ovulation and progesterone and estrogen production. (See the chapter on ovaries for more information.)

GH promotes an increase in the size and number of all cells in the body capable of growth and reproduction. It stimulates protein synthesis and muscle growth while stimulating the body to use up fat stores. It increases blood sugar levels (thus stimulating insulin production) by decreasing carbohydrate utilization. It also stimulates the production of a substance that promotes proper bone and cartilage growth, development, and repair. Growth hormone is also necessary for tissue repair, and plays a role in increasing our resistance to disease by stimulating the immune system. It can speed wound healing, decrease blood urea levels, and prevent or reverse osteoporosis. It is released in response to sleep, fasting and exercise. Growth hormone levels generally decline with age.

Prolactin aids in mammary gland growth during pregnancy and later initiates milk production by the glands after birth. Prolactin formation is normally inhibited until pregnancy and it reaches a maximum after giving birth.

The posterior pituitary secretes oxytocin and antidiuretic hormone (ADH, also known as vasopressin). Oxytocin is actually produced by the hypothalamus but stored in the posterior pituitary. It enhances uterine contractions once the onset of labor has begun and also causes milk to travel from the alveoli to the ducts of the mammary gland, making it available for the nursing child.

ADH is also produced in the hypothalamus and stored in the posterior pituitary. It controls the permeability of the renal tubules. Secretion of ADH causes the kidneys to conserve water and electrolytes. ADH is inhibited by both alcohol and caffeine, which is why they both lead to dehydration.

Symptoms of Pituitary Malfunction

1) Any symptoms listed in the chapters for adrenals, thyroid, testes, and ovaries, can be from pituitary malfunction causing hormonal disturbances involving those organs.

2) General symptoms of anterior pituitary imbalance can include neck and head pain on the left side, chronic headaches at the level of the eyes, and seizures, especially at night.

3) Over production of ACTH (possibly due to low blood sugar) can indirectly cause increased levels of aldosterone and estrogen causing water retention, dysmenorrhea, edema, weakness and hypertension. It can also lead to hyperglycemia and possibly non-insulin dependent diabetes. Other symptoms include glucose intolerance and personality changes. Chronic over production and resultant over production of cortisol will shrink thymus and lymphatic tissue, and decrease formation of antibodies and sensitized lymphocytes, thus greatly decreasing immunity.

4) Under production of ACTH can cause adrenal cortex atrophy, hypoglycemia, generalized weakness, low blood pressure, salt loss and increased skin pigmentation. Intolerance to stress and infection will also result.

5) Over production of TSH can lead to hyperthyroidism with symptoms such as personality changes, irritability and increased sweating. Under production of TSH will cause hypothyroidism.

6) Over production of FSH and LH will cause early sexual maturation and acne. Under production can cause gonadal atrophy, infertility, amenorrhea, decreased sperm production and impotence.

7) Over production of GH (GH can increase 10 fold from hypoglycemia or prolonged fasting) can cause diabetes by stimulating insulin production until the beta cells "burn out". It can also produce gigantism or acromegaly.

8) Under production of GH can lead to weak ligaments and tendons, decreased rate of wound healing, hypoglycemia, dwarfism and poor bone development.

9) Under production of ADH can cause diabetes insipidus and excessive urination, dehydration.

10) Over production of ADH can lead to edema and hypertension.

11) In endocrine disorders, new symptoms can crop up as the body tries to correct itself. To give a fictitious example - a woman is suffering from hypoadrenia due to bad diet and stress in her home life. Her

pituitary will step up ACTH production to try to increase cortisol production. Since the adrenals are depleted, the ovaries will somewhat increase production of estrogen since it too is a steroid and they have a few functions in common. The increased estrogen production causes the thyroid to slow down. The woman develops menstrual cramping and starts putting on weight. The point of this scenario is to show the interrelationship within the endocrine system and how in most cases three or four glands will require treatment before normal function is restored.

Causes of Pituitary Malfunction

1) It has been shown that our cranial bones as well as sacrum and coccyx move very slightly in response to breathing. It is theorized that this movement helps to "pump" the pituitary and pineal glands and that if these movements are abnormally altered, one result can be pituitary malfunction. I have clinically confirmed this many times as have other chiropractors and osteopaths. Restoring biomechanical equilibrium to these structures can bring dramatic clinical results if it is the cause of the problem. The following can cause a dysfunction in the normal biomechanics: being delivered by forceps or other birth trauma, whiplash (due to attachments of sternocleidomastoid and trapezius to the cranium), improper breathing, injury or trauma to the head, long dental procedures (due to drilling, mouth props etc. this is very common). Wearing tight helmets, carrying weight on your head and dental occlusion causing an imbalance of forces to be transmitted through the mandible to the temporal bone and the rest of the cranium, can also cause cranial malfunction and pituitary disturbance.

2) Other malfunctioning endocrine glands can alter pituitary outflow and lead to malfunction (make sure the ovaries, testes, adrenals and thyroid are working properly).

3) Dr. Pavlo Airola feels that mental and physical sexual stimulation too early in life, as well as a high consumption of meat, dairy, sugar, salt, alcohol, tobacco and caffeine can over stimulate the pituitary.

4) Severe emotional trauma can alter pituitary function.

5) Concentrated sweets will cause abnormal blood sugar disturbances and thus altered ACTH and TSH output.

6) Julian De Vries in *Contraceptive Pill Criticized* feels that birth control pills will increase your risk of pituitary cancer.

7) Cortisone medication can cause decreased ACTH production.

8) Hypoglycemia and prolonged fasting can lead to over production of growth hormone and eventual exhaustion of production.

9) Rich fatty meals suppress GH production as does cortisone and epinephrine containing medications.

10) Nicotine causes over production of ADH while alcohol and caffeine suppress ADH production (that is why beer makes you urinate so much).

11) We have seen that heavy metal toxicity can alter pituitary function.

12) Exposure to extreme cold without proper clothing can decrease the size of the pituitary. It will also lead to an increase in TSH and ACTH production, which could eventually exhaust it.

Prevention and Treatment of Pituitary Malfunction

1) Occasionally, spinal misalignment in the cervical spine needs to be corrected in pituitary cases. Also seeing someone trained in cranial manipulation can be very helpful. Often a good chiropractor or osteopath can do both.

2) Rubbing a reflex point right between the eyebrows (the glabella) is often helpful. Try twice a week, one minute each time.

3) Stay away from rich fatty foods, alcohol, tobacco, caffeine, concentrated sweets, medications containing epinephrine and cortisol (do not stop any medications without a doctor's supervision).

4) Foods high in lecithin may be helpful. The pituitary is composed partially of lecithin.

5) Avoid excessive sexual stimulation especially from TV, novels, etc.

6) Dressing warmly, going to bed early, exercising, and positive thoughts all help balance GH and ACTH production.

7) It is accepted by many that being outdoors (especially on a sunny day) without glasses or contacts will stimulate and aid pituitary function as it does the pineal.

8) Taking gonadotropins (LH or FSH) as medication should be looked at and studied particularly with a holistically oriented physician before it is undertaken. It should be avoided if possible. Side effects can include ovarian enlargement, multiple births, blood clots and depression.

9) Synthetic oxytocin is used to induce early delivery, in second trimester abortions, and to control postpartum bleeding. Side effects have included uterine rupture, fetal and maternal death, vomiting, cardiac arrhythmia and neonatal jaundice.

Supplement Recommendations

SUPREME NUTRITION PRODUCTS

1) Endo Supreme

Chapter 5:   OVARIES

Anatomy and Physiology

The ovaries are two almond shaped glands each about 1 1/4" long with a combined weight of about 1/4 ounce. At puberty, a female has about 400,000 egg cells of which about 450 mature in one's life. The ovaries are composed of thousands of follicles, each of which contains an immature egg.

In this chapter we will discuss the menstrual cycle as well as functions of estrogen, progesterone, LH and FSH.

Estrogen is a steroid compound (made from cholesterol) secreted by the ovarian follicles, corpus luteum, the adrenals and, during pregnancy, by the placenta. Estrogen performs the following functions during puberty:

1) Growth of the uterus, fallopian tubes, vagina, endometrium, ovaries and breasts (and aids in developing them into milk producing organs)
2) Growth of bones, closing of epiphyses and broadening of pelvis
3) Deposition of fat in thighs and gluteal region
4) Increases synthesis of protein

Estrogen (after puberty) also causes hypertrophy of the uterus, sodium and water retention, and inhibition of LH and FSH secretion.

Progesterone is produced by the corpus luteum (we are discussing it here instead of in the uterus chapter due to its interactions with estrogen, FSH and LH), adrenal cortex and placenta (during pregnancy). Progesterone prepares the fallopian tube to supply nutrients to the fertilized egg and prepares the uterus for implantation of the egg. It also contributes in developing the breasts as milk secreting organs. Progesterone can block the effects of estrogen, and estrogen can inhibit progesterone. Large quantities of progesterone can inhibit LH and FSH. The thyroid gland may in some way regulate progesterone production also. The liver deactivates or degrades excess estrogen and progesterone.

The menstrual cycle has two main functions: to release a mature egg and prepare the uterus for its implantation.

Following menstruation, FSH is secreted from the anterior pituitary. This leads to growth and maturation of the egg which produces estrogen. Estrogen secretion increases until it peaks about 1-2 days before ovulation. The estrogen peak is followed by a surge in LH secretion and a doubling of FSH secretion. This causes final growth, swelling and then rupture of the follicle, and the egg is released. The follicle then forms the corpus luteum (due to influence of LH).

During the second half of the cycle (post ovulation), estrogen and progesterone levels rise for the first 7-10 days. This rise inhibits both LH and FSH, thus preventing any more eggs from maturing during this cycle. The estrogen and progesterone prepare the uterus for implantation of the fertilized egg. Progesterone causes swelling, increased blood flow and nutrient storage in the endometrium.

If no egg has been fertilized by about the 22nd or 23rd day, progesterone and estrogen secretion starts to decrease and the corpus luteum begins to degenerate. As degeneration continues, estrogen and progesterone continue to decrease and FSH and LH begin to rise. The corpus luteum degenerates by about the 26th day. Loss of hormonal stimulation causes the outer layers of endometrial tissue to die and blood seeps in. After approximately 28 days, the outer tissue layers separate from the uterus and cause contraction to expel the uterine contents; menstruation begins. Meanwhile the increase in FSH and LH levels are beginning egg maturation for the next cycle.

Symptoms of Ovarian Dysfunction

Most symptoms of ovarian dysfunction before menopause are related to improper ratios of estrogen as compared with progesterone. Any menstrual pain at all is not normal and is a signal of some dysfunction in the body.

If there is too much estrogen secretion in relation to progesterone, the woman's flow will be heavy and last up to 7 days. Water retention, breast soreness and cramping will be likely and the cycle will usually be less than

28 days.

If there is too much progesterone in relation to estrogen, the flow will be light and can last only 1-2 days. Water retention and cramps will be rare and the cycle will last 30-40 days.

The ideal is much closer to this latter description than to the over secretion of estrogen.

Symptoms of dysmenorrhea and premenstrual tension can include depression, tension, cramping (very severe at times), water retention, backaches, breast tenderness, fainting spells, nausea, vomiting, diarrhea and irregular cycles. Some very severe cases are bedridden the first few days of each period.

Menopause is the time in a woman's life when menstruation ceases. It should be a relatively easy transition. Signs of abnormal menopause and possible dysfunction (usually adrenal or pituitary dysfunction also contribute) include: numbness, heart palpitations, hot flashes, chills, sweats, headaches, insomnia, depression, pelvic pain and mental instability.

Causes of Ovarian Dysfunction

1) Pituitary malfunction causing an imbalance in ovarian hormone secretion (usually from increased ACTH, FSH or LH)
2) Spinal misalignment in the lumbar spine or sacral area
3) Liver sluggishness and not breaking down excess ovarian hormones (especially estrogen). This can also happen from eating or being exposed to too many phytoestrogens (plants with estrogen like compounds) or xenoestrogens (chemicals with estrogen like compounds). Phytoestrogen containing foods (amounts will vary) include: soybeans, certain other beans, flax, sesame seeds, wheat, fenugreek, oats, barley, yams, rice, alfalfa, apples, carrots, pomegranates, hops, fennel and anise. Xenoestrogens can be found in many chemical compounds. Bisphenol A, found in some plastics, is one major source of xenoestrogens.
4) X-rays without properly shielding the ovaries
5) Not enough sunlight. Sunlight regulates melatonin production. (See

the pineal chapter.) Imbalances in melatonin production can retard ovulation and delay sexual maturation.

6) Pain due to ileocecal valve syndrome can be misdiagnosed as right ovarian pain.

7) Hypoadrenia can cause estrogen/progesterone imbalance.

8) Causes of Dysmenorrhea
   a. Adrenal, pineal or thyroid dysfunction
   b. Calcium deficiency: can be due to decreased assimilation, thyroid or parathyroid imbalance or too high a protein intake causing increased calcium excretion.
   c. Chilling of extremities due to improper clothing, too tight waist bands, etc.
   d. Mental stress (due to its effect on adrenals, pituitary, and thyroid)
   e. Uterine malposition
   f. Constipation and ileocecal valve syndrome will aggravate dysmenorrhea
   g. Spinal and pelvic misalignment, especially if back pain accompanies it

9) Causes of amenorrhea can be: anemia, anorexia, protein deficiency which can be due to hypochlorhydria (see the stomach chapter) or due to blood sugar handling problems, hyperthyroidism, adrenal malfunction and obesity. Amenorrhea after pregnancy, miscarriage or abortion should be examined by a gynecologist.

10) Causes of difficult menopause: as menopause approaches, properly functioning adrenal glands should produce enough estrogen to make the transition symptom free. If hypoadrenia is present, the pituitary will increase production of ACTH and FSH, which will exhaust the adrenals even more, causing the autonomic nervous system to cause the symptoms we previously listed.

Other Indications of Ovarian Dysfunction

1) Check indications of adrenal malfunction to see if the problem is secondary to hypoadrenia.

2) To see if calcium deficiency exists put a blood pressure cuff on your leg and inflate it to about 80mm. Hg pressure. Leave it on for 4 minutes and if your muscle cramps, it is a good indication of a possible calcium deficiency. Remember if there is a deficiency in calcium, it is probably due to either too many protein or oxalic acid

containing foods in your diet, thyroid or parathyroid imbalance, or poor assimilation (decreased hydrochloric acid secretion). It is less often due to a deficiency in your diet itself. Correct the cause. If you take calcium, calcium citrate or citramate is much preferred to calcium carbonate.

Prevention and Treatment of Ovarian Dysfunction

1) We have seen that correcting dysbiosis and eliminating foods you are sensitive to often go a long way towards correcting problems concerning hormone imbalances. At the same time, eliminate xenoestrogens from your diet. In correcting dysbiosis, remember that sexual partners need to be checked and treated also.
2) Have a good chiropractor check for spinal misalignments and correct them.
3) Follow the instructions in the liver chapter and get lots of sunshine.
4) Get out in the sun (to regulate melatonin), follow a whole foods diet, get ample exercise and avoid sexually stimulating books, TV shows and movies. This will help keep hormone production regular.
5) For dysmenorrhea: avoid mustard, vinegar, sugar, tobacco, caffeine and chocolate. Eliminate intake of trans fats and decrease salt intake.
6) Make sure your liver is functioning properly, especially if you suffer from dysmenorrheal. A B vitamin deficiency or toxic bowel can overtax the liver and decrease its ability to break down estrogen.
7) Try to trace the problem back to its cause; remember malfunctioning adrenals, thyroid, and pituitary, can all lead to an imbalance of ovarian hormones.
8) If you suspect a calcium deficiency, try lowering your protein intake, make sure your hydrochloric acid secretion is adequate (see the stomach chapter) and eat lots of dark greens (broccoli, kale, etc., not high oxalic acid greens like spinach and chard).
9) Dropped uterus, ileocecal valve syndrome, food allergies and constipation can all aggravate premenstrual symptoms. Correct these conditions if they exist. (See their respective chapters.)
10) Try a pure seaweed supplement like Alaria Supreme to help regulate ovarian hormones.
11) Try supplements that help strengthen the liver (see liver chapter) as they may help break down excess hormones and normalize cycles. Wear loose clothing and don't overeat. Get enough sleep. A 20-minute hot foot and leg bath (113°F), a warm enema at onset of

menses, or a heating pad on the abdomen (for up to a few hours) will help relieve the pain. The following herb teas may reduce symptoms and overcome dysmenorrhea: catnip, peppermint, sorrel, shave grass, plantain, red raspberry leaf, crampbark, yarrow, amaranth, and red sage.

12) Premenstrual edema can be helped by minimizing salt intake and eating a lot of garlic, watermelon and cucumber. Also, add vigorous exercise to your routine.

13) Chamomile tea and aloe vera juice can help bring on a late period.

14) Sassafras tea is reported to help in cases of amenorrhea.

15) For a difficult menopause, fix your adrenal glands if they are malfunctioning, get lots of outdoor exercise (3-5 hours daily), try a 20-minute 110°F hot sitz bath and get lots of sleep. A 30-minute neutral bath daily can help relieve symptoms. The following herbal teas are reported helpful for difficult menopause: licorice root, elder, unicorn root, black cohosh, and sarsaparilla (all contain natural estrogens).

16) Stay on the adrenal recovery diet. (See the adrenal chapter.) Also, eating foods high in natural plant sterols will ease the transition. These include sesame seeds, sunflower seeds, rice bran, chestnuts, potatoes, tomatoes, eggplant, pepper, barley, and peas (women with premenstrual symptoms of increased estrogen listed in the symptoms section of this chapter may benefit by avoiding these foods).

17) Phytoestrogen supplements like THORNE RESEARCH'S Metabalance can often be helpful. We have mixed feelings about bio-identical hormones. They have helped many women though we have seen side effects like back pain that couldn't be resolved until the patient stopped taking them. We have seen good results in patients prescribed natural plant extracts from the company Bezwecken. Ask your alternative medicine physician about them.

18) Rubbing the following reflex points for 2 minutes every other day for 8 days can help restore normal ovarian function. The points are located on the anterior part of the pubic bone (one point on each side).

One patient had a four-year-old son, and had been trying unsuccessfully for three years to have a second child. She was found to have hypoadrenia, pituitary-cranial malfunction and ovarian disturbances. We put her on the adrenal recovery diet, rubbed the adrenal and ovarian reflex areas, and fixed the cranial malfunction, and within three months she became pregnant and has since given birth to a healthy child. This is one of many similar cases. I never know what to say when a female patient comes in saying "Thanks for helping me get pregnant".

Supplements Recommendations

THORNE RESEARCH:

1) Meta-balance

2) Basic B Complex

3) SAT

4) TAPS

SUPREME NUTRITION:

5) Endo Supreme

6) Body Guard Supreme

7) Wild Greens Supreme

LuRONG LIVING:

8) LuRong Essential

Michael Lebowitz DC and Ami Kapadia MD

Chapter 6: **TESTES**

Anatomy and Physiology

The testes are two glands suspended within a sac of skin called the scrotum. They are composed of a large number of seminiferous tubules. The testes have two main functions: formation, development and excretion of sperm (occur in seminiferous tubules) and secretion of testosterone.

FSH from the anterior pituitary stimulates the creation and development of sperm. Sperm consist of a head, neck, body and tail. The nuclear material in the head is responsible for fertilizing the egg. Sperm formation starts when a boy is approximately 13 years old. They need a temperature of 95° to develop properly and that is why they are located outside the main body cavity. The smooth muscle in the wall of the scrotum can somewhat regulate temperature by contracting and bringing the testes closer to the body when cold and relaxing when too warm. Sperm continue to mature and are stored in the epididymis, which rests on the posterior surface of the testes, and in the vas deferens and its ampulla. Each ml of semen will contain on the average 120,000,000 sperm and since the average ejaculation is 3.5ml, it contains about 400,000,000 sperm.

LH secreted from the anterior pituitary stimulates testosterone production and secretion by the interstitial cells of Leydig. These cells make up 20% of the mass of the adult male testes.

Testosterone can be synthesized from cholesterol and is present in males and females, though in much larger quantities in males. In puberty, testosterone has the following functions:

1) Causes growth of the penis, scrotum, testes, and prostate
2) Causes growth of facial, axillary, pubic, leg, and arm hair
3) Enlarges the larynx and deepens the voice
4) Increases skin thickness, protein production, ligamentous growth, muscular development, and bone thickness
5) Increases deposition of calcium salts in bone and closing of bony

epiphyses

The adrenal glands also produce testosterone. Production decreases after age forty but continues throughout life. It is broken down in the liver and its byproducts are excreted in the urine and feces.

Symptoms of Testes Dysfunction

1) Infertility due to decreased number of sperm
2) Poor muscle and ligamentous development
3) Brittle bones

Causes of Testes Dysfunction

1) Improperly working pituitary gland (see the pituitary chapter.)
2) Overworked liver being unable to break down excess testosterone. (See the liver chapter to learn how it gets overtaxed.)
3) Not dressing warmly enough in cold weather can cause the testes to decrease in size by 50%. If this becomes a habit it could cause dysfunction.
4) Wearing pants or underwear that are too tight, or taking very hot baths, can increase testicular temperature and retard sperm development.
5) Hypothyroidism and hypoadrenia have been shown to alter testicular function.
6) Low back and colon x-rays without shielding the testes can possibly injure them.
7) Spinal misalignment in the lumbar and sacral areas
8) In animal experiments, taking epinephrine (which humans sometimes have prescribed in acute allergy attacks and as an ingredient in pain injections) will decrease sperm development, reduce sex drive, and cause degenerative changes in the seminiferous tubules.

Prevention and Treatment of Testes Dysfunction

1) Check for pituitary, adrenal, thyroid, and liver dysfunction and correct them as needed. (See their respective chapters.)
2) Make sure the testes are properly shielded during x-rays.
3) The same reflex points listed in ovary treatment #18 are good for the

testes.

4) If sciatica or low back pain is also present see a good chiropractor to correct any spinal misalignment.

5) Dress warmly and don't wear clothing that is too tight.

6) Avoid tobacco, alcohol and caffeine. Minimize sugar intake and avoid epinephrine type drugs if possible.

7) A cold compress for 5 minutes followed by a hot compress for 10 minutes and another cold compress for 5 minutes once daily applied to either the lumbar spine or inner thighs is reported to stimulate testicular function.

8) Sunlight striking the scrotum and penis will stimulate testosterone production. Sunlight "is beneficial in general, but it's especially helpful when it strikes these areas.

9) For impotence, try THORNE RESEARCH's Perfusia and LuRong Living's LuRong Essential which may also increase libido. L-Tyrosine can also increase libido.

10) Chickweed and/or mullein in poultice form is supposed to aid swollen testes.

11) Testosterone is sometimes given as a medication to treat eunichism, impotence and general testosterone deficiency states. It is sometimes used in post menopausal women as part of hormone replacement. We are hesitant to endorse these uses as there can be potential side effects and it might suppress the small amount you may still be producing.

Supplement Recommendations

THORNE RESEARCH

1) Perfusia

2) Zinc Picolinate

3) L-Tyrosine

SUPREME NUTRITION

4) Endo Supreme

5) LuRong Essential

Chapter 7: **THYMUS**

Anatomy and Physiology

The thymus gland is a pink-grey organ that lies underneath the top of the breastbone. In animals, it is known as the sweetbreads. Sometimes the pancreas is also called the sweetbreads.

No one knew much about the thymus gland until the last 50 years or so. On autopsies, it was noticed that young adults that had died in traumatic accidents often had much larger thymus glands than those dying from diseases of a chronic nature, and it was also believed that the thymus ceased to function after childhood.

It is now known that the thymus gland is largest and most active in the neonatal and pre-adolescent periods and begins to regress in adulthood. Precursor cells from bone marrow migrate to the thymus where they mature into white blood cells called T-cells or T-lymphocytes. These T-lymphocytes govern cellular immunity, which means that they help cells recognize and destroy invading bacteria, virus, fungi, etc., as well as abnormal cell growth such as cancer and foreign tissue. They may also help prevent auto-immune conditions. There are various types of T-lymphocytes and other thymus secretions that are beyond the scope of this book.

Experiments done on animals have shown that if the thymus is removed before birth, the baby will accept an organ transplant without rejecting it (it has lost its ability to recognize foreign tissue). At the same time that baby will exhibit little or no ability to fight off disease or infection. Animals that had their thymus removed would develop cancer rapidly upon injection of cancer cells into their body, while animals with an intact thymus would in most cases destroy the cells. Overall, it has been shown that the thymus plays a crucial role in the development of a normal, competent immune system.

Symptoms of Thymus Dysfunction

A person with an underactive thymus gland will be prone to getting sick often. Infection will be common and will often be chronic and prolonged. Allergies will also be more likely. Other symptoms include swollen glands, depression, extreme sweating and puffiness of the throat. The person will be a likely candidate for cancer and possibly auto-immune disease.

Causes of Thymus Dysfunction

1) We talked in the adrenal chapter about how cortisol taken in the form of hydrocortisone medication, or having an over productive adrenal gland, will cause the thymus and lymphatic tissue to shrink and cause an underactive thymus. The most common causes of too much cortisol production are mental stress and eating large amounts of sweets (for other causes of increased cortisol production and side effects of cortisone medication see the adrenal gland chapter).
2) Many times following organ transplant surgery, glucocorticoids are injected to inhibit the immune response so our bodies won't have the ability to recognize and reject the foreign tissue.
3) Chronic or severe acute diseases can overtax the thymus and cause it to temporarily shrink in size.
4) Exposure to toxic chemicals/metals can also shrink thymus tissue.
5) Spinal misalignment in the cervical spine can cause thymus malfunction.
6) Refined foods (sugar, oil, etc.), alcohol, caffeine, tobacco and marijuana, all depress thymus function via increased production of cortisol.
7) X-rays striking the thymus can decrease thymus function.
8) Adequate amounts of growth hormone are necessary for development and function of the thymus. An improperly functioning pituitary can thus alter thymus function. (See the pituitary chapter.) Also, an overactive pituitary secreting too much ACTH will cause over secretion of cortisol and shrink thymus tissue.

Prevention and Treatment of Thymus Dysfunction

1) Avoid caffeine, tobacco, alcohol, marijuana, refined sweets and refined fats. Also avoid foods you are sensitive to.
2) Make sure during chest and dental x-rays that your thymus is

shielded.

3) Proper sleep, exercise, a whole foods diet and keeping your stress level down will help keep the adrenals and the thymus functioning properly.

4) Correct any pituitary or adrenal malfunction that may be occurring. (See their respective chapters.)

5) Chronic dysbiosis can weaken the thymus over time. (See the dysbiosis chapter.) Have this checked and corrected.

6) If you suspect any spinal misalignment, see a good chiropractor.

7) Avoid exposure to heavy chemicals and pesticides as much as possible.

8) Rubbing a reflex point at the level of the nipple underneath the axilla (bilaterally) vigorously for two minutes daily for one week will be helpful. Also, percussing (tapping) on the breast-bone over the thymus one minute daily will help stimulate it.

9) Avoid medications and ointments containing hydrocortisone if possible.

10) Bee propolis seems to have a strengthening effect on the thymus gland and the immune system in general. I have found that many times if children chew two propolis tablets hourly at the first signs of a flu or ear infection it won't come on. Morinda Supreme also has many times aborted an oncoming cold.

Supplement Recommendations

THORNE RESEARCH

1) Im-Encap

SUPREME NUTRITION PRODUCTS

2) Thera Supreme

3) Morinda Supreme

Chapter 8: **PARATHYROID GLANDS**

Anatomy and Physiology

There are four small parathyroid glands located just behind the thyroid, (two on each side). Each is approximately 6mm long, 3mm wide, and 2mm thick.

The parathyroid gland produces a hormone known as parathyroid hormone. Parathyroid hormone secretion is stimulated when blood calcium levels are low and is inhibited when blood calcium levels are high. Parathyroid hormone has the following effects:

1) Promotes kidney formation of the active metabolite of vitamin D, thus aiding in calcium absorption
2) Activates and increases the number of osteoclasts, thus increasing the rate of bone destruction and making calcium and phosphorus available
3) Delays formation of osteoblasts (bone forming cells)
4) Increases absorption of calcium and phosphate by the small intestine
5) Increases reabsorption of calcium and excretion of phosphate by the kidneys. Phosphate is important in maintaining our body's acid-alkaline balance and helps in regulating carbohydrate digestion.

Parathyroid hormone, calcitriol, and vitamin D are our body's principal regulators of calcium and phosphorus balance. Without enough vitamin D, the effects of parathyroid hormone are decreased.

A decrease in serum calcium will stimulate parathyroid hormone activity and cause hypertrophy of the parathyroid (common in rickets, pregnancy, and lactation).

Too much serum calcium causes decreased activity and shrinking of the parathyroid.

Symptoms of Parathyroid Dysfunction

1) An under functioning parathyroid gland may cause any of the following symptoms: muscle tension, cramps, neurotic behavior, susceptibility to allergies, cataracts (excess calcium deposits in tissues), dry rough skin, tingling around the mouth and extremities, alkaline gut (with associated symptoms of emaciation, burping, constipation, hemorrhoids, stiff joints), and hypertension.
2) An over functioning parathyroid gland may cause any of the following symptoms: weakness, weak bones, nausea, kidney stones, increased urination, and depression.

Causes of Parathyroid Dysfunction

1) A chronically low serum calcium level due to poor diet or bad assimilation (especially decreased hydrochloric acid output) can cause hypertrophy and eventual exhaustion of these small glands.
2) Lack of exercise leads to bone resorption and increased serum calcium levels, thus inhibiting parathyroid function. Taking too many calcium or vitamin D supplements can have similar effects.
3) Spinal misalignment in the mid-cervical spine can possibly cause parathyroid dysfunction.

Prevention and Treatment of Parathyroid Dysfunction

1) Vigorously rub a reflex point in the belly of the teres minor muscle, halfway up the outside border of the scapula for 1 minute daily, for one week.
2) For an under functioning parathyroid, get lots of sunshine for vitamin D production (and consider vitamin D supplementation if you live in an area without much sunshine or are consistently using lotion or sunscreen), eat calcium rich foods (seeds, dark green vegetables like kale, collards and dairy if it isn't a sensitivity for you). Lots of exercise will also increase bone growth, decrease serum calcium and stimulate parathyroid function.
3) For an over functioning parathyroid, consider avoiding calcium and vitamin D supplements.
4) Have a good chiropractor check for spinal misalignment and correct it.

Supplement Recommendations

THORNE RESEARCH

    1) Calcium Citrate

    2) Calcium Citramate

    3) D-1000

    4) D-5000

    5) Vit D/K2

Michael Lebowitz DC and Ami Kapadia MD

Chapter 9:   **PINEAL GLAND**

Anatomy and Physiology

The pineal gland is a small gland located inside the skull. It is richer in lecithin than any other part of the body and we are just now beginning to understand some of its functions.

It appears that the major function of the pineal is to produce serotonin and melatonin. Serotonin is converted into melatonin in the pineal. We will be discussing melatonin here (for more on serotonin see the neurotransmitter chapter). Melatonin is produced in greater quantities during darkness, as the pineal gland is inhibited by light. Melatonin is known to influence the menstrual cycle and other body rhythms, sexual maturity, and pigment changes.

It seems that the natural cycles of daylight and darkness produced by the sun causes the body to produce the right amount of melatonin and that too much or too little can be problematic.

It is felt by many that the pineal gland is tied to endocrine function and may actually be the master endocrine gland, instead of the pituitary or hypothalamus. Pineal tumors bring on early puberty. Epinephrine in increased amounts can stimulate melatonin production. Melatonin is formed from the amino acid Tryptophan in a multi-step cycle that first forms serotonin.

Many Americans over 50 years old have calcified pineal glands. It has been suggested that lower levels of melatonin (associated with calcified pineal glands) may be associated with higher rates of certain types of cancers. No one knows for sure why the pineal calcifies, but it has been shown that in countries where people eat a higher percentage of unrefined food and spend more time outdoors, the incidences of calcified pineal glands are much less common.

Causes of Pineal Dysfunction

1) Cranial dysfunction (see causes of pituitary gland malfunction #1) can cause secretory changes in pineal output. This can happen from head trauma, dental visits, car accidents etc.
2) Too much artificial light and wearing tinted glasses may upset pineal function. It is theorized that light striking the retina will send signals to the pineal via neurotransmitters and that sunlight is ideal, while the spectrum of artificial light and light passing through glass is changed and may alter pineal function.
3) Stress, refined sugars, and other factors that increase epinephrine output (as well as epinephrine medications) will increase melatonin production and, if chronic, cause pineal dysfunction.
4) People that work nights or stay up late and don't get outside much during the daylight hours won't inhibit pineal secretions and this will overtax the pineal gland. Even a brightly lit room has only a fraction of the light that is present in outdoor sunlight.
5) Too high of an exposure to electromagnetic fields, especially during sleep, can decrease melatonin production. Ideally, have nothing plugged in within six feet of your head while you sleep.

Symptoms of Pineal Dysfunction

1) Any symptoms that increase with sleep may be due to pineal dysfunction. Menstrual problems, breast soreness, craving alcohol and many symptoms of dysfunction of the other endocrine glands may be secondary to pineal dysfunction. Panic attacks have also been linked to melatonin deficiency, as has increased cancer risk.

Prevention and Treatment of Pineal Dysfunction

1) Don't wear sunglasses during the day. Make sure your room is totally dark when you sleep at night.
2) Go to sleep early (between 9pm and 10pm is ideal), keep regular hours and get plenty of natural sunlight.
3) Eat foods high in lecithin.
4) Don't take epinephrine containing medication and keep stress and refined sweets intake to a minimum.
5) Have an Applied Kinesiologist or another expert in cranial imbalances check for cranial dysfunction and spinal misalignment.

6) Minimize exposure to electromagnetic fields, especially at night.
7) Taking melatonin supplementation may bring relief but may further suppress the body's own manufacturing of melatonin. It might be better to try L-Tryptophan with Pyridoxal-5-Phosphate or 5-Hydroxytryptophan.

Supplement Recommendations

THORNE RESEARCH

    1) L-Tryptophan

    2) 5-Hydroxytryptophan

    3) Pyridoxal-5-Phosphate

SUPREME NUTRITION PRODUCTS

    4) Body Guard Supreme

    5) Endo Supreme

    6) Ashwaganda Supreme

Michael Lebowitz DC and Ami Kapadia MD

Chapter 10:   **LIVER**

Anatomy and Physiology

The liver is a large reddish-brown organ located in the upper right part of the abdominal cavity. It weighs about three pounds and is approximately 3-5% fat. It performs over 500 functions.

You could function fairly normally with as little as 1/6th of your liver intact, and if as much as 80% of your liver were cut away it would grow back to a full size in approximately three months. Because the liver is designed in this way, it is usually hard to determine if the liver is damaged until the damage is quite advanced.

Some of the major liver functions include:

1) Synthesizes 1-2 grams of cholesterol daily (about three times the average daily dietary intake) to be used to produce steroid hormones and bile salts
2) Stores vitamins A, B-12, D, K, and iron
3) Synthesizes blood proteins - albumin, globulin, and fibrinogen (as well as other clotting factors)
4) Converts dietary fatty acids into circulating phospholipids
5) Converts beta-carotene to Vitamin A
6) Stores up to 1 liter of extra blood in times of excess blood volume and supplies it to the body when needed (e.g. in times of blood loss or heavy exercise)
7) Converts up to 1/2 ounce of alcohol per hour into carbon dioxide and water
8) Makes 1 quart of bile daily to aid in dietary fat emulsification
9) Detoxifies incompletely digested proteins, excess hormones (estrogen, progesterone, testosterone, etc.), drugs, food additives, poisons, etc.
10) Converts glucose, pyruvic acid, amino acids, glycerol and lactic acid to glycogen. It can store up to 4 ounces of glycogen to be released when it is needed to maintain blood sugar levels, upon signals via epinephrine or glucagon.

11) Stores sodium, which aids in neutralizing some toxins
12) Uses bile salts to aid in breakdown and absorption of vitamins A, D, E, and K
13) Takes ammonia which is formed from the breakdown of protein and changes it into urea for kidney excretion
14) The kupffer cells of the liver filter out about 99% of the bacteria in the blood coming from the intestines before it can enter the general circulation
15) Breaks down lipids for energy, desaturates fatty acids
16) Forms new sugar (gluconeogenesis). Cortisol can increase this process up to 1000% and greatly increase blood sugar levels. The liver can synthesize up to 4 ounces of glucose daily and will do this during fasting and diabetes mellitus. A properly functioning liver will buffer or tone down swings in blood sugar by up to 65%.

Bile from the liver is either stored in the gallbladder or secreted into the duodenum. It is approximately 97.5% water, 1.1% bile salts, and has small amounts of bilirubin (a byproduct of used and ruptured red blood cells), cholesterol, lecithin, and electrolytes (especially sodium and chloride ions). The bile salts decrease the surface tension of fat particles in the small intestine, allowing them to be broken down into smaller pieces so they can be acted upon by lipase. Without bile salts, only about half the fat eaten would be absorbed as compared to 97% with normal bile secretion.

Symptoms of Liver Dysfunction

1) Any symptom due to an excessive amount of hormones, be it estrogen, testosterone, cortisol, etc., could be due to a malfunction in the secreting organ or could be due to an overtaxed or sluggish liver being unable to degrade it.
2) Increased cholesterol levels can be from overproduction by the liver.
3) Abdominal bloating, tenderness over the liver area
4) Acne, skin rashes, photophobia, constipation, itching, fatigue, loss of appetite, yellow tinge to skin (due to excessive bilirubin), bitter or metallic taste in the mouth, split ends, brittle nails, all may indicate liver dysfunction.
5) Symptoms of hypothyroidism can be due to excess estrogen in the blood, due to the liver not breaking it down.
6) Blood sugar handling problems due to the glucose-glycogen-glucose

conversion. Large swings in blood sugar can be due to a diseased liver.

7) Liver congestion can cause portal hypertension leading to pressure in the venous system, thus causing hemorrhoids or varicose veins.

8) Pain between the shoulder blades, inability to digest fats properly, and decreased resistance to infection can all indicate liver dysfunction.

9) Swelling in legs due to an overtaxed liver being unable to destroy extra antidiuretic hormone.

10) People with a large number of food allergies almost always have some type of subclinical liver dysfunction.

Causes of Liver Dysfunction

1) It is up to the liver to detoxify most poisons (chemicals, metals, food toxins, etc.) we eat, touch, smell, and breathe daily. In my practice, it seemed like the liver would reach a saturation point in some patients and then cause symptoms. To give an example, a good friend of mine is a carpenter and is constantly exposed to toxic chemicals used to treat lumber. His liver is working very hard to break these down. When his diet was high in fatty foods - corn chips, vegetable oil, peanut butter, and other fried foods, he would break out in a skin rash and hemorrhoids. His liver didn't seem to be able to handle both the chemicals and the fatty foods. We worked on his liver reflex points and eliminated the "bad fats" from his diet and his symptoms cleared up. A few months later his diet temporarily slipped and his symptoms returned until he began to abstain again.

2) Fried foods, fats from grain-fed animals, hydrogenated vegetable fat (margarine, etc.), too much vegetable oil, and roasted nuts, can overtax and congest the liver.

3) Polluted air and water, certain prescription medications, strong cleaning solutions, soaps, deodorants, birth control pills, pesticides, herbicides, food additives, etc., can overtax the liver and damage it.

4) Dysbiosis (the organism itself and the bio-toxins it produces), eating foods you are sensitive to, and toxic metals all greatly overtax the liver.

5) Spinal misalignment in the mid thoracics can cause liver dysfunction.

6) Tannic acid (in tea), and BHA (a common food additive) have been implicated in liver cancer.

7) Caffeine and other methylxanthines can greatly overwork your liver. (See the chapter on food sensitivities/toxins.)

8) Any dysfunction in any of the other organs of elimination - colon, kidneys, lungs, and skin, can overload the liver by giving it more work to do.

9) Artificial sweeteners have been implicated in liver damage.

10) Diets too high in protein can overwork the liver (converting excess ammonia to urea).

11) Refined sugar can damage mitochondria in liver cells and decrease the ability of the liver to break down excess triglycerides causing elevated triglyceride and cholesterol levels.

12) Alcohol is a well known cause of liver cirrhosis. Tobacco and recreational drugs must also be detoxified by the liver and can overwork it.

13) Corticosteroids (cortisone etc.), carbon tetrachloride, alcohol and tetracycline can all cause triglyceride and fat buildup in the liver.

14) A B vitamin deficiency can make the liver unable to break down excess steroid hormones.

15) A major cause of liver dysfunction is a toxic bowel (often secondary to dysbiosis) with a resultant increase in transit time. This overworks the kupffer cells and other parts of the liver causing liver congestion and sluggishness.

16) Due to the liver's role in venous pressure, if inflating a blood pressure cuff around your calf to 180mm Hg pressure causes muscle pain, it is often due to liver congestion. This test can also be used to monitor your progress.

Prevention and Treatment of Liver Dysfunction

1) It is necessary to figure out and eliminate all food allergies/food toxins. (See the chapter on food allergies/food toxins.)

2) It is necessary to find and treat all chronic, subclinical infections. (See the chapter on dysbiosis.)

3) Beets, black radish and dark greens are all very cleansing for the liver. The juice of 1/2 of a large beet daily will help (more can be too cleansing and cause nausea).

4) The juice of 1/2 of a lemon in a glass of warm water upon rising every morning will also help cleanse the liver.

5) Fried foods, roasted nuts, peanut butter, vegetable oil, margarine and grain fed meat should all be abstained from as should alcohol, tobacco, caffeine, chocolate and non-essential medications (if possible—this should only be done under supervision of physician).

Also, keep sugar and concentrated sweets to a minimum. Keep this up strictly for 3 months.

6) Drink a lot of water and get plenty of exercise and sunshine to help stimulate the channels of elimination.

7) Live where the air and water are clean. Try to avoid sprayed foods, harsh cleansers, deodorants, food additives, cosmetics, etc.

8) If you have pain between the shoulder blades, or have a sitting job or bad posture, see a good chiropractor to check for spinal misalignment.

9) Rub a reflex area on the right side between the 5th and 6th ribs from under the nipple to the sternum. Do this for 1 minute, every other day, for 2 weeks.

10) In infants with neonatal jaundice, sunlight, a full spectrum artificial light, or blue light will bring dramatic results. In conjunction with this, Takesumi will also help. Put 1 teaspoon of Takesumi in a cup of water, strain it, and then fill your baby's bottle with the water. Sunlight and Takesumi, due to their detoxifying properties, are also helpful in adult liver disorders.

11) For breaking up liver congestion, dip a piece of flannel or cotton in warm castor oil, set it on the liver and cover it with plastic. Secure it in place and use overnight. Do this three times over two weeks.

12) I have found that a fairly deep massage over the liver area below the ribs will help stimulate and cleanse a sluggish liver.

Supplement Recommendations

SUPREME NUTRITION

1) Body Guard Supreme

2) Wild Greens Supreme

3) Thera Supreme

4) Takesumi Supreme

THORNE RESEARCH

5) TAPS

6) SAT

7) Phosphatidyl Choline

Chapter 11:   **GALLBLADDER**

Anatomy and Physiology

The gallbladder is a small organ, located next to the liver that stores and concentrates bile. It has a storage capacity of 40-70ml., and by absorption of water, salts, and electrolytes through the gallbladder mucosa, the bile becomes between 4-12 times more concentrated than it was in the liver.

Bile is composed of water, salts, fatty acids, cholesterol, lecithin, bilirubin, and mucus. The liver makes about one quart of bile daily and whatever isn't sent directly to the duodenum to emulsify fat is diverted to the gallbladder and stored until needed.

When fat from a meal reaches the duodenum, cholecystokinin and secretin are secreted into circulation. These hormones stimulate contraction of the gallbladder. This contraction plus peristalsis in the small intestine causes the Sphincter of Oddi to relax and the bile then enters the duodenum. With a fairly fatty meal, the gallbladder can completely empty within one hour.

Symptoms of Gallbladder Dysfunction

Approximately 500,000 people in the U.S. each year are hospitalized due to gallbladder problems and it is estimated that 20% of the population over 40 years old has gallstones.

Symptoms that may indicate gallbladder disturbance and/or stones include pain (very severe at times) under the right lower ribs possibly extending to the right shoulder, vomiting, bloating and gas (especially after a fatty meal), cold sweats, belching, food intolerance and jaundice.

Causes of Gallbladder Dysfunction

1) Not drinking enough water and not exercising enough can cause gallbladder disturbances.
2) Spinal misalignment in the mid thoracic spine. This can be due to poor

posture, too many one-handed sports (tennis, ping pong, etc.) trauma, etc.

3) Some authorities feel that holding in your anger can cause gallbladder or liver problems.

4) Gallstones form when the bile becomes saturated with cholesterol; some of this cholesterol precipitates out and hardens (90% of all gallstones are cholesterol). The following substances can lead to increased cholesterol buildup and have been implicated as possible gallstone causes: birth control pills, refined starches (white flour, white rice), sugar, fatty meat, greasy or highly seasoned foods, corn oil, dairy products and high protein foods in excess.

5) People with diabetes, gallbladder cancers and liver diseases suffer from an increased incidence of gallstones.

6) A weak immune system (thymus, spleen, etc.) can increase the likelihood of infection in the gallbladder epithelium. An infection here will cause the mucosa to absorb more water and electrolytes. As a result, cholesterol will over saturate the bile, drop out, and form stones.

7) As with most other organ systems, dysbiosis, food sensitivities and toxic metals and chemicals can play a role. (See their respective chapters.)

Prevention and Treatment of Gallbladder Dysfunction

1) Correct dysbiosis, food sensitivities and toxic metals. (See their respective chapters.)

2) Exercise will increase gallbladder emptying and drinking water will dilute the bile. Lots of both are good preventative measures.

3) Treatments in the liver chapter will often help the gallbladder as well.

4) Pears, parsley, comfrey tea, and cascara sagrada tea, are all reported to help poorly functioning gallbladders.

5) Make sure your liver is functioning correctly as well as your small intestine. (See their respective chapters.)

6) "Primitive" societies whose diets are almost totally composed of whole unrefined foods have extremely low incidences of gallstones.

7) Put a hot fomentation over the gallbladder for 15 minutes followed by rubbing the area for 2 minutes with ice. Repeat three times. This may help dislodge stones. Do it once daily for 1 week.

8) Take grapefruit and/or orange rind (from unsprayed fruit only), boil it for 20 minutes and drink 3 glasses of the tea daily. This is reported to

help gallbladder problems.

9) The same reflex areas listed for liver treatment are beneficial for the gallbladder.

Supplement Recommendations

THORNE RESEARCH

1) LipoTrepein

SUPREME NUTRITION PRODUCTS

2) Body Guard Supreme is an herb that has been traditionally used for centuries in people with gall stones. Again, it is always wise to consult your physician to discuss supplementation.

Chapter 12:　　　　　**STOMACH**

Anatomy and Physiology

The stomach is a major protein-digesting organ made up of the cardia, fundus, body and pylorus. It has a capacity to hold 2-3 quarts of liquid or solid material at a time, secretes up to 2 1/2 quarts of digestive juices daily, and has a normal pH between 1.5-3. There are about 35 million glands in the stomach. Stomach secretions include pepsin, hydrochloric acid, mucus, a small amount of lipase (a fat digesting enzyme), gastrin and intrinsic factor.

The stomach has two types of glands. The gastric glands have mucus neck cells (which secrete mucus), parietal cells and chief cells. The parietal cells secrete hydrochloric acid (HCl) which has a pH of 0.8. Many people, as they get older, slowly lose their ability to produce enough HCl. There is a lot of evidence that this is not a normal condition but a result of years of abusing their stomach (so it just begins to quit). The chief cells secrete a protein digesting enzyme called pepsin. Pepsin works best in a pH of around 2 and if the stomach pH gets as high as five (fairly common in people on antacids), it will be inactivated. HCl helps activate pepsin by lowering the stomach pH. Pepsin is necessary to digest the collagen in meat and without pepsin meat digestion will be significantly retarded.

Three main factors cause the stomach to secrete HCl and pepsin:

1) Food entering the stomach causes release of gastrin. Via circulation, the gastrin will reach the gastric glands and cause them to increase pepsin production three fold and HCl eight fold.
2) Stimulation from the vagus nerve increases gastric secretion - pepsin more than HCl.
3) Smelling food and possibly even strong thoughts of food will stimulate gastric secretion.

The second type of gland in the stomach is the pyloric gland. It secretes a thin mucosal layer to protect the stomach wall from being digested by HCl and pepsin. Other mucus cells produce an alkaline gel-like mucus for added protection and to help lubricate the food. Any irritation in the stomach will increase mucus production even more. Without mucus, it would take about three hours for the HCl and pepsin to eat a hole in the stomach wall.

Intrinsic factor secreted in the stomach combines with vitamin B-12 and aids in its absorption in the ileum of the small intestine. Most cases of vitamin B-12 deficiency are due to lack of intrinsic factor and the resulting failure of B-12 to be assimilated rather than from dietary deficiencies.

The fundus has very little tone and mainly holds food. If there is already older food in the stomach, when new food enters, the old food will be positioned nearer the stomach walls. The gastric glands will start secreting, and about 3 times a minute a peristaltic mixing wave will help mix the food and gastric gland secretions, and move the outermost layer of food toward the antrum. In the antrum, gastric secretion is increased and the peristaltic waves are up to six times stronger. This greatly increases the mixing and digestion of the food (the food-gastric gland mixture is called chyme and will be referred to as that from this point on). From the antrum, the chyme is moved toward the pyloric sphincter, which is kept constricted to stop chyme from entering the duodenum of the small intestine prematurely. Only a strong peristaltic wave will push chyme through.

Certain factors will increase the tone of the pyloric sphincter and slow stomach emptying. These include:

1) When the pH of the chyme is below 3.5-4.0 in the duodenum (this slowing is accomplished through a reflex known as the enterogastric reflex via the vagus nerve).
2) Fatty food or distention due to too much chyme in the duodenum will also produce an enterogastric reflex.
3) Products that irritate the duodenal lining will produce an enterogastric reflex.

Increased acidity, fats, and irritants will also cause the small intestine to secrete secretin and cholecystokinin. These hormones decrease stomach secretions, thus slowing stomach emptying.

If the stomach has been empty for at least eight hours, it can produce a strong contraction that we call "hunger pangs". These will last between 2-10 minutes and will increase our desire to eat.

Studies have shown that an average meal, if entering an empty stomach, can take up to four hours to totally pass through into the duodenum. If eating in between meals is practiced, some of that original meal can stick around for a longer time in the stomach. Eating in between meals may encourage fermentation, putrefaction and gas.

Symptoms of Stomach Dysfunction

Throughout the rest of this chapter we will mainly be concentrating on three major conditions that affect the stomach: too little HCl secretion, too much HCl secretion and hiatal hernia syndrome. For information on H.Pylori, read the small intestine chapter.

1) Hypochlorhydria (too little HCl secretion) is a diagnosis that is often overlooked by the medical profession, but I, among others, have found this to be a fairly widespread condition with many consequences. Symptoms of decreased HCl (hypochlorhydria) can include: odiferous gas, stomach distention shortly after eating, a burning feeling in the stomach 1-3 hours after eating sometimes accompanied by a headache, gallstones, problems digesting protein, rectal itching and decreased assimilation of iron, copper, zinc, manganese, and magnesium (deficiencies of these minerals can lead to prostate problems, slow ligament and muscle healing, heart problems, food sensitivities, muscle cramps, heart palpitations, etc.).

2) The hydrochloric acid in the stomach kills many germs that enter our body through our food. Hypochlorhydria can result in more of these germs, causing illness. Decreased HCl will also make calcium assimilation very difficult (see the parathyroid chapter for low calcium symptoms); and if the lack of acidity is systemic (throughout the body), calcium will tend to be taken out of solution and deposited in joints and connective tissue (causing arthritis, bursitis, etc.). In addition, partially digested protein due to hypochlorhydria can enter the circulation and cause inflammation and antigen activity. The antigen activity and decreased calcium assimilation make allergies a common symptom of hypochlorhydria.

3) Interestingly enough, hypochlorhydria will respond to taking antacids.

The antacids will make the stomach even more alkaline and this will stimulate the body to produce HCl which will digest the protein and stop the heartburn. The habitual taking of antacids will exhaust the stomach's ability to produce HCl.

4) Symptoms of too much HCl and possibly ulcers are: burning pain on an empty stomach, pain that is relieved by eating, and vomiting blood.

5) Hiatal hernia is a partial protrusion of the stomach above the diaphragm. This is another condition that is sometimes missed by medical diagnosis. Symptoms include heartburn that can radiate to the chest and mimic pains of an oncoming heart attack, burping, vomiting, feeling like your food isn't going down and indigestion after a heavy meal.

Causes of Stomach Dysfunction

1) General causes of stomach dysfunction include eating too many refined foods or greasy foods, not chewing well, overeating, too many different food combinations at a meal, alcohol, spicy foods, and caffeine.

2) Eating a heavy protein and starch or sugar at the same meal (e.g. a hamburger on a bun). As the stomach works on the protein, the carbohydrate is waiting. If stomach emptying is delayed (from overeating, eating in between meals, etc.), the carbohydrate can start to ferment and cause heartburn and organic acid formation. At this point, an antacid is often taken. This will neutralize the organic acid and relieve the heartburn, but will also neutralize the HCl and retard the protein digestion.

3) Too much salt intake and cigarette smoking both lead to increased incidence of stomach cancer.

4) Spinal misalignment in the mid thoracics can cause stomach dysfunction.

5) Causes of hypochlorhydria:

   a) Eating foods that are too cold or drinking cold or ice water before or with your meal

   b) Taking antacids fairly regularly, through acid rebound, will exhaust the parietal cells and cause hypochlorhydria.

   c) B vitamin deficiencies (due to poor diet, increased intake of sweets, etc.)

d) Stress will cause increased sympathetic nervous system stimulation and hypochlorhydria.

e) Eating in between meals or eating a diet too high in protein will eventually exhaust the parietal cells.

f) I have found that eating foods you have an allergy or food sensitivity to will decrease HCl production in the long run as will certain forms of dysbiosis.

6) Causes of increased HCl and/or ulcers (through other mechanisms) include:

   a) stress (via excessive vagal stimulation)
   b) smoking
   c) overly spicy foods
   d) hypoadrenia
   e) certain medications (aspirin, non-steroidal anti-inflammatory medication, prednisone, cortisone, and reserpine).

7) Causes of hiatal hernia include overeating or too many combinations at one meal (this leads to stomach distention and gas and can push the stomach through the diaphragm). Laying down and resting or bending over after a large meal can have similar results. Tight belts, corsets, lack of exercise and trauma to the stomach can all lead to hiatal hernia. People with weak diaphragms (especially due to poor breathing habits) are more prone to hiatal hernia. In my practice, I have found this condition common in pregnant women in their second or third trimesters. They will often come in weak and pale and complain of no appetite and an inability to hold food down.

8) According to Guyton's *Basic Human Physiology*: "Gastric ulcers occur in patients who have normal or LOW secretion of HCl....ulceration in the stomach almost certainly results from reduced resistance of the stomach mucosa to digestion rather than to excess secretion of gastric juice." He goes on to state that aspirin and alcohol reduce mucosal resistance and can contribute to this.

Prevention and Treatment of Stomach Dysfunction

1) Chew well, don't eat in between meals, don't eat more than three different courses per meal, and avoid tobacco, excessive salt, overly spicy foods and caffeine. Eat when relaxed.

2) Vigorously rub a reflex area between the 5th and 6th, and 6th and 7th ribs, on the left side from directly under the nipple to the sternum, for one minute, 3 times a week, will help many stomach problems.

3) Treat H.Pylori if appropriate. (See the small intestine chapter.)

4) Ingesting milk if allergic/sensitive to it may cause the pyloric sphincter to spasm. Ingesting any food you're allergic/sensitive to may temporarily halt HCl secretion (or cause over secretion) or just irritate the stomach in general.

5) See a good chiropractor to check for spinal misalignment. Applied Kinesiologists have also found that certain cranial misalignments may contribute to hypochlorhydria.

6) Animal studies have shown that charcoal broiled foods, smoked foods, and cayenne pepper can cause stomach cancer in susceptible individuals.

7) Exercise can reduce stress and thus balance stomach secretions.

8) Hot and cold applications (3 minutes hot followed by 30 seconds cold repeated 3 times, twice daily, over the stomach and mid thoracics) can help regulate the stomach.

9) The following herbs are reported helpful for stomach dysfunction in general: slippery elm, red clover, chickweed, yarrow and strawberry leaves.

10) For a bleeding stomach - put an ice pack over the stomach, swallow small amounts of ice, don't eat and call your doctor immediately.

11) For hypochlorhydria:

a) See a chiropractor skilled in Applied Kinesiology and cranial correction.

b) Drink a glass of warm water 15 minutes before each meal, OR put an ice pack over the stomach for 10 minutes, 15 minutes before the meal.

c) Make sure your B vitamin intake is optimal.

d) Don't overeat high protein foods and avoid antacids.

e) Don't eat in between meals.

f) Making a tea from the rind of sour oranges and drinking it before meals is helpful to restore normal HCl secretion.

g) Sunlight tends to normalize HCl secretions.

12) For hyperchlorhydria and ulcers:

a) Drink a glass of ice water 15 minutes before your meals.

b) Eat lots of olives, millet, avocados, and almonds.

c) Avoid antacids, milk, overly spicy foods, and high protein foods.

d) Don't eat in between meals.

e) Drink lots of water, decrease stress, exercise, and get lots of sun.

f) Eating aloe vera gel is often helpful as is burdock root tea.

g) Eating refined sugar can increase stomach acidity by 20% and aggravate ulcers.

h) Taking hydrochloric acid may help temporarily but it is better (if possible) to get the body to produce the right amount by dealing with causes.

13) For hiatal hernia syndrome:

a) To prevent it: don't overeat, don't bend over too soon after eating, no eating in between meals or late at night, practice deep breathing and eat lots of high fiber foods.

b) See an Applied Kinesiologist or other health care practitioner trained in physically correcting the condition with soft tissue manipulation. The results can be instantaneous in some cases. Follow up this correction by drinking 16 oz. of water daily on arising (while standing up) waiting 5 seconds and then doing a vertical jump. Often the stomach loses its "structural correction" during sleep and this can often correct it. Do this for 2 weeks while the diaphragm heals up and strengthens.

14) Many antacids contain aluminum hydroxide. Aluminum is a suspected cause in Alzheimer's disease and can also cause weakness, constipation, and phosphorus deficiencies. Antacids containing magnesium hydroxide can cause diarrhea, iron and potassium deficiencies.

Supplement Recommendations

SUPREME NUTRITION PRODUCTS

1) Wild Greens Supreme

Chapter 13:   Small Intestine

Anatomy and Physiology

The small intestine is the largest part of the gastrointestinal tract and is composed of the duodenum (which is about 1 foot long) jejunum (5-8 feet long) and ileum (6-12 feet long).

The duodenum is the major portion of the small intestine where enzyme secretion takes place. The small intestine secretes sucrase (breaks sucrose into glucose and fructose); maltase (breaks maltose into glucose); and lactase (breaks lactose into glucose and galactose; lactase is missing in a good percentage of people). It also secretes peptidase to split peptides (from protein) into amino acids, and lipase to break down fat into glycerol and fatty acids.

The duodenum receives bile from the liver and gallbladder to decrease the surface tension between the large fat globules and water, and break them into smaller globules that can be acted upon by lipase. Lipase, amylase, trypsin, chymotrypsin and sodium bicarbonate are received from the pancreas upon hormonal signals from pancreozymin and other hormones (produced in the small intestine) and neural signals from the vagus nerve.

Epithelial cells in the small intestine secrete over 1/2 gallon of a neutral fluid daily to supply a watery substance to mix with the chyme and provide a substance to aid in electrolyte and vitamin absorption through the villi.

Brunner's glands in the duodenum secrete mucus in response to secretin, vagal stimulation and direct stimulation of food in the small intestine. This mucus protects the duodenal wall from the digestive juices. Goblet cells in the mucosa also produce mucus. In general, the duodenum isn't as well protected with mucus as is the stomach and is more prone to ulcers. A deficiency of pancreatic juices to neutralize the acidic chyme from the stomach, or stress causing sympathetic inhibition of enzyme secretion can lead to duodenal ulcer formation.

Approximately 1/2 of your carbohydrate digestion is performed by amylase from the pancreas, 40% from the saliva and 10% from intestinal amylase. Ninety-five percent of your fat digestion is performed by pancreatic lipase and 5% from intestinal and lingual lipase.

The small intestine is covered with villi and microvilli. They increase the surface area of the intestinal wall exposed to chyme by 60,000%. The increased surface area makes the small intestine very efficient in absorption. Capillaries in the villi absorb amino acids, glucose, fructose and galactose, while lacteals absorb fatty acids and glycerol to travel through the lymphatic vessels.

As chyme enters the small intestine, the acidity of it causes secretion of the hormone secretin, which signals the pancreas to secrete alkaline juices to neutralize the chyme. The chyme also initiates a type of small intestine contraction known as segmentation, which helps to mix and chop the chyme and propel it along. These contractions occur about once every 5 seconds in the duodenum but only half as fast in the ileum. Peristaltic waves also occur and aid in chyme propulsion. It takes about 2-3 minutes for the chyme to advance 1 inch, and all together food can remain in the small intestine between 3-10 hours normally. Eating and stomach distention both can increase peristalsis in the small intestine. Harmful irritants reaching the small intestine can initiate what is called a peristaltic rush, which can empty the entire small intestine into the colon within a few minutes. Food you are allergic to can also do this and lead to diarrhea due to the lack of time for fluid absorption.

Symptoms of Small Intestine Dysfunction

1) General symptoms of small intestine dysfunction include abdominal bloating and pain, gas, diarrhea, and nausea.
2) Lactase deficiency can cause gas, nausea, bloating, cramps, diarrhea, asthma and congestion when dairy products are ingested.
3) Many feel that congestion in the lacteals and lymphatics of the small intestine contributes to narcolepsy.
4) Symptoms of duodenal ulcers include midmorning and middle of the night pain relieved by eating. The pain lasts for 1-3 weeks at a time and then subsides.

Causes of Small Intestine Dysfunction

1) Some causes of small intestine dysfunction are primarily related to the liver, pancreas, gallbladder, and stomach, all affecting digestion in the small intestine. The correct cause must be determined.
2) Spinal misalignment in the lower thoracics can affect small intestine function.
3) As with most gastro-intestinal issues, dysbiosis and food sensitivities are a major cause of dysfunction and must be addressed. (See respective chapters.)
4) Antibiotic therapy can kill off helpful bacteria in the small and large intestine and can cause an alkaline gut where harmful gas producing bacteria will proliferate. Lack of HCl will contribute to this also.
5) Certain spices, alcohol and caffeine can cause irritation and a resultant over-secretion of mucus in the small intestine. This can "plug" the villi and decrease vitamin and mineral absorption leading to various deficiencies. In this case, even a healthy diet won't be assimilated properly.
6) Causes of duodenal ulcers:

    a) H. Pylori- a bacteria often found in poultry and eggs is a major cause of ulcers.
    b) Increased HCl secretion in the stomach up to 1500% of the normal amount. (See stomach chapter for causes.)
    c) Stress causing increased sympathetic nerve flow and decreasing secretion of mucus from Brunner's Glands.
    d) An overworked pancreas from overeating, eating between meals, etc. and, not secreting enough bicarbonate.

7) Eating any food you're sensitive or intolerant to can cause disturbances in the small intestine.

Prevention and Treatment of Small Intestine Dysfunction

1) Diagnose and treat dysbiosis and food sensitivities.
2) Avoid overly spicy food, caffeine, alcohol and refined carbohydrates (sugar, white flour, white rice) so you won't over secrete mucus and decrease your absorption.
3) Make sure your liver, pancreas, gallbladder, and stomach are functioning properly. (See their respective chapters.)

4) Eat lots of raw fruit and vegetables (raw and/or cultured) to promote growth of healthful bacteria.

5) Treat H. pylori if present. Melia Supreme, Golden Thread Supreme, and SF734 can all be effective remedies. Poultry and eggs must be avoided during this time. After treatment, only eat poultry and eggs at home and wash all the surfaces they touch before they are cooked. Wash your hands after touching raw poultry and eggs to prevent contamination (and possible re-infection). You should also make sure you cook them thoroughly.

6) For intestinal gas, try a scoop of Takesumi Supreme in water.

7) Slippery elm tea is reported to be beneficial for inflammation of the small intestine.

8) See a good chiropractor if you believe spinal misalignment to be a contributing cause.

9) Two bilateral reflex areas are helpful. The first is located along the border of the 8th-11th ribs and cartilage. The second is along the upper third of the thigh half way between the front and inside. Both should be vigorously rubbed for 1 minute every other day. In cases of narcolepsy or Crohn's disease, do it twice daily for 3 minutes.

10) For duodenal ulcers try 4 ounces of fresh raw cabbage juice 4 times daily and drink lots of water. Decrease your stress level. Sugar should be avoided.

11) If you have eaten too many irritating foods and suspect your villi to be "plugged" and your absorption decreased, the following may be helpful. You can try increasing your intake of raw papaya and pineapple and you can also try periodic juice fasting (juice fasting longer than 3 days should only be done under the supervision of a physician who is knowledgeable about this modality of detoxification).

Also 30 minutes before each meal take 1/2 scoop of Takesumi supreme to "scrub" out the mucus. If there is mucus in you stool from this treatment, don't be concerned.

Supplement Recommendation

-For H. Pylori

THORNE RESEARCH

1) SF734

SUPREME NUTRITION PRODUCTS

2) Melia Supreme

3) Golden Thread Supreme

-In general

THORNE RESEARCH

1) L-Glutamine

SUPREME NUTRITION PRODUCTS

2) Takesumi Supreme

Chapter 14:   ILEOCECAL VALVE

Anatomy and Physiology

Although the ileocecal valve isn't an organ or gland, it can cause a myriad of symptoms and the medical profession often misses correct diagnosis of ileocecal valve syndrome. Knowing the function, symptoms, and problems relating to this valve might save someone much invasive and expensive testing.

The ileocecal valve is at the very end of the small intestine (ileum) and connects it to the first part of the large intestine (the cecum). If you draw a line from your umbilicus to your right anterior superior iliac spine (the most prominent part of your pelvis in the front of your body), the valve would be located just below the midpoint of that line.

The ileocecal valve has two main functions. The first is to prevent the backflow of fecal contents from the colon to the small intestine. The second is to prevent the contents of the ileum from passing into the cecum prematurely.

Gastrin is a hormone produced when food is in the stomach. When the chyme with gastrin approaches the valve, the gastrin causes it to relax. Also, following a meal, the gastroileal reflex will open the valve to let the chyme through. At other times, the valve remains shut. Irritation and/or distention of the cecum will keep the valve tightly constricted.

Symptoms of Ileocecal Valve Syndrome

The main problems that can affect the valve are that it can become "stuck open" or it can become spastic. Symptoms that can occur with either condition include pain in the area of the valve (can be mistaken for right ovary pain), dizziness, low back pain, shoulder pain (mainly on the right side), nausea, faintness, paleness, sudden thirst, bad breath and ribbon like stools. Ileocecal valve syndrome will also aggravate dysmenorrhea and endometriosis and should be evaluated in these conditions.

1) People with valves "stuck open" usually suffer from loose bowels, get overly emotional, and exhibit vitamin C deficiencies (their vitamin C is exhausted detoxifying the backflow of fecal material).
2) People with spastic valves tend to be constipated.
3) In my practice when I have seen cases of diarrhea caused by this condition, closing the valve would stop the diarrhea immediately.

Causes of Ileocecal Valve Syndrome

1) Any chronic irritation in the area of the cecum such as an irritated appendix (from too much spicy, greasy, or refined food, not enough exercise, water, or any other unhealthy practice that will clog the lymphatic system) can cause the valve to spasm.
2) Alcohol, caffeine, carbonated beverages, chocolate, incomplete digestion (from not chewing well, eating too frequently, overeating, dysfunction of the stomach or small intestine, etc.) can cause dysfunction of the valve.
3) Any irritation in the small intestine, eating too frequently, strong emotional upset, or overeating a food you're sensitive or intolerant to can cause the valve to become "stuck" open.
4) Eating refined sweets, especially if you have blood sugar handling problems, can make the valve get stuck open, and eating sweets after correcting valve problems can cause its recurrence.
5) Spinal misalignment in the upper lumbar spine can cause ileocecal valve syndrome.
6) Fecal contents with a pH under 6.8 tend to distend the colon by making it atonic, causing the valve to become spastic. Conversely, fecal contents too alkaline (pH over 7.0) will make the colon hypertonic and relax the valve.
7) A hyper or hypotonic psoas muscle can contribute to ileocecal valve syndrome.
8) Intestinal dysbiosis can cause ileocecal valve problems.
9) A magnesium deficiency can cause the valve to be "spastic".

Prevention and Treatment of Ileocecal Valve Syndrome

1) Avoid foods you are sensitive to and correct dysbiosis. (See their respective chapters.)
2) Avoid overly spicy food, alcohol, and caffeine. Don't overeat.
3) Rubbing a reflex area on the front of the right shoulder (where the

biceps muscle goes through a groove in the humerus) for one minute every other day for two weeks will be helpful.

4) Go to a good chiropractor to check for spinal misalignment as a possible cause.

5) If stuck open, press straight down (over the valve) through the body during five successive expirations, use 3-4 pounds pressure and let up on inspiration. If spastic, press down through and toward the left shoulder for five successive expirations. An Applied Kinesiologist will know how to do this if you would prefer professional treatment.

6) If your valve was stuck open, put a cold plastic bag of water over the valve for twenty minutes before bed daily for one week to help prevent recurrence.

7) An open ileocecal valve should not always be closed. If you ate an irritating substance, your body in its wisdom may have opened the valve to get the harmful substance through faster. Go over the dietary history of the past two days before deciding on treatment.

8) If the valve is spastic, try taking 1 Magnesium Citrate capsule with each meal.

Supplement Recommendations

THORNE RESEARCH

1) Magnesium Citrate

Chapter 15: **LARGE INTESTINE**

Anatomy and Physiology

The large intestine is about five feet long and composed of the cecum, ascending colon, hepatic flexure, transverse colon, splenic flexure, descending colon, sigmoid and rectum.

The large intestine has no villi and produces no digestive enzymes. It does secrete mucus to help the digested food along and hold the fecal material together. It also plays a role in protecting the walls of the large intestine from bacterial activity and neutralizes some of the fecal acids. Between 1/3-1 quart of water, electrolytes, and some vitamins, are absorbed daily through the colon. If colon bacteria are normal, they produce vitamins B-1, B-2, B-12 and K, and all with the possible exception of B-12 are absorbed and used by the body traveling first to the liver via portal circulation. Absorption and storing fecal material are the large intestine's two main functions.

After chyme enters the large intestine, much absorption occurs in the cecum and ascending colon. Mixing movements occur every few minutes and last about one minute apiece. The chyme is rolled and mixed to expose most of it to the colon's surface for absorption. Over 80% of the material reaching the large intestine is reabsorbed. There are no peristaltic waves in the colon but a few times daily (usually after meals) a segment of the colon will constrict (usually in the transverse or descending colon). This will occur twice in close proximity to force the fecal material along. Upon the fecal material reaching the rectum, a parasympathetic reflex is set up to cause defecation to occur.

The external sphincter is under voluntary control and we can mentally overcome this reflex and prevent defecation if we so desire.

Feces are usually 75% water, 7-8% dead bacteria, 2-7% fat, .5-1% protein, 5-10% roughage, byproducts, digestive juices, etc.

Symptoms of Large Intestine Dysfunction

1) If the bowel is overworked or malfunctioning, the body will try to find other areas of elimination, thus infections, skin problems, congestion, etc., can all be symptoms.

2) Diarrhea (frequent passage of watery bowel movements), constipation (difficult, infrequent defecation), increased cholesterol levels, cystitis, gallstones and appendicitis can all be due to toxic bowels.

3) Diverticula (small herniations through the muscular wall of the colon) are symptoms of colon dysfunction. If they inflame it is called diverticulitis and symptoms can include pain, tenderness, diarrhea or constipation and fever.

4) Colitis or inflammation of the colon is marked by fever, weight loss, weakness, abdominal pain and/or diarrhea.

5) An imbalance in colon flora can manifest as a burning pain somewhere in the body, especially the feet.

6) Hemorrhoids are actually varicose veins in the rectal area and can cause pain, itching, bleeding and distention upon straining to defecate. They can be secondary to liver or adrenal dysfunction.

7) Slow transit time: If your transit time is over 36 hours, you may have a colon problem (or it could be elsewhere in the gastrointestinal tract). To check your transit time, take 2 scoops of Takesumi Supreme before a meal and record the time you ingested it. Watch your feces and record the time the last of the Takesumi Supreme passes through (it will cause black stools). The time between ingestion and the last bit leaving is your transit time. After you've been treating your colon for 1-2 months you may want to recheck and see if it has improved.

Causes of Large Intestine Dysfunction

1) Dysbiosis and food sensitivities are the most common source of bowel dysfunction and can lead to "leaky gut", IBS, constipation, diarrhea, gas, abdominal pain, etc. (See respective chapters for more detail.)

2) Slow transit time can cause colon dysfunction. Ideally, food that enters your body should pass through within 24-36 hours. If food remains in the gastrointestinal tract for a longer period of time, gas, putrefaction and fermentation can set in. Causes of slow transit time can be lack of adequate fiber in the diet, not drinking enough water,

eating in between meals, magnesium deficiency, and eating too many refined foods. A diet low in roughage and high in refined carbohydrates can also cause: diverticula to form (the feces are hardened and the extra strain to move them causes the out pocketing), constipation and bacterial changes (due to the fermentation and putrefaction). People in "primitive" societies on diets of unrefined foods exhibit very low incidences of colon problems.

3) People on a high fiber diet most often have lactobacillus and streptococcus as their main intestinal flora. On a low fiber diet, E. coli proliferate (especially if your refined carbohydrate intake - white flour, white sugar, etc., is high) and can lead to diverticulitis, cystitis, appendicitis and gallbladder inflammation. Taking antibiotics can also change the bacterial flora for the worse.

4) In a colon with slowed transit time, bacterial imbalance and low roughage, bile acids can be converted into carcinogenic substances once they reach the colon. Staying in contact with the colon walls for long periods of time, these substances could possibly increase the risk of colon cancer. One of the bile acid breakdown products (lithocholate) that can be formed also signals the liver to decrease bile acid production. Since cholesterol is used to synthesize bile acids, a decreased synthesis will raise cholesterol levels and also increase susceptibility to gallstones.

5) Causes of colitis include: dysbiosis, hypoadrenia, a weak immune system, hypochlorhydria, decreased roughage, increased use of refined carbohydrates, stress, antibiotics and eating foods you're sensitive to (see the adrenal, thymus, and stomach chapters for more information).

6) Besides an imbalance in intestinal flora, a high fat intake is correlated to a high incidence of colon cancer. This includes refined animal and vegetable fat. When exposed to air, meat fat can form malonaldehyde, which can be related to an increased risk for colon cancer.

7) Spinal misalignment in the lumbar spine can cause colon dysfunction.

8) Hemorrhoids can be caused by a congested liver, hypoadrenia, and a low fiber, high-refined carbohydrate diet.

9) If your stomach or small intestine is malfunctioning or you don't chew well, and partially undigested food reaches the colon, it will putrefy and could damage the colon as a result.

10) Diarrhea can be a sign of colon dysfunction. It can also be due to

eating something you're sensitive to, a stuck open ileocecal valve, vitamin B deficiency, taking too much magnesium, and medication side effects. It could also be your body's effort to flush through a harmful substance as quickly as possible.

11) Constipation can injure the colon or be a sign of a malfunctioning colon. Causes include: dysbiosis, magnesium deficiency, a low roughage diet, sensitivity to dairy (or other food sensitivities), wearing restrictive clothing, not drinking enough water, lack of exercise, chronic use of laxatives exhausting bowel tone, spastic ileocecal valve, excess worry, and side effect of certain medications. Voluntarily inhibiting your external sphincter muscle too often, to prevent defecation, can cause constipation and retard the reflex, leading to an atonic colon. Establishing regularity is very important in preventing constipation. The thyroid, adrenals, liver and parathyroid should also be evaluated in cases of constipation as possible causes.

Prevention and Treatment of Large Intestine Dysfunction

1) Correct dysbiosis and avoid foods you are sensitive to. (See their respective chapters.) This is the most important step.

2) Eat a diet composed of mainly unrefined foods (whole grains, fruits, vegetables, beans, nuts, and seeds), drink at least 6 glasses of water daily, and get lots of exercise. Avoid caffeine, alcohol, overly spicy food, greasy food, margarine and refined sugar.

3) Stay off all dairy for one month and see if your condition improves.

4) Evaluate and treat, if necessary, your liver, thyroid, adrenals, stomach and small intestine. All can affect your colon.

5) Chew your food well; don't drink fluids with your meals.

6) The following herbs are reportedly healing and tonic to the colon: mullein, sumac berries, slippery elm and red raspberry leaves.

7) If you suspect spinal misalignment is affecting your colon (especially if you suffer from low back pain) see a good chiropractor.

8) One reflex area is extremely helpful in colon problems. The whole outside of the thigh (right and left) should be rubbed vigorously daily for two weeks. When you find particularly tender areas, spend a little extra time on them.

9) In cases of colitis, check for dysbiosis, food sensitivities, hypoadrenia, hypochlorhydria, and decreased thymus function. Stay on the adrenal recovery diet for one month.

10) A heating pad over the bowel can often relieve pain there.

11) In cases of diarrhea, find the cause. To relieve symptoms, a hot half bath is helpful as is an enema. Eating unrefined carob or chewing on a guava leaf can also relieve diarrhea.

12) Eating a high roughage, low refined carbohydrate diet will do much for constipation. Other helpful remedies include:

    a) Massaging the colon - start at the cecum and go up the ascending colon, across the transverse, and down the descending colon. This can help loosen hardened fecal material.

    b) Magnesium citrate, 3 or more caps daily, will usually correct constipation.

    c) Drink enough water (6-8 glasses daily) and get lots of exercise.

    d) Evaluate your liver, thyroid, ileocecal valve and parathyroid for possible involvement.

    e) A warm or hot compress to the abdomen or a hot sitz bath can be helpful in relieving constipation.

    f) Try to develop regularity in bowel habits and don't inhibit the natural urge to defecate whenever possible.

13) Senna is a very strong laxative and its use should be discouraged. Cascara sagrada is reported to tone the bowels as well as act as a safe laxative and when withdrawn, the bowels should continue to work fine due to its tonic effect.

14) For leaky gut, after dysbiosis is corrected, try supplementing with a good probiotic as well as L-Glutamine.

Habitual use of stimulating laxatives tends to decrease bowel tone and create a laxative dependency. Their use should be avoided.

Many anti-diarrhea drugs have possible dangerous side effects such as numbness of extremities, depression, headaches, vomiting and increased heart rate. Again, seek out the cause and try to naturally restore the body to proper functioning.

Supplement Recommendations

THORNE RESEARCH

1) L-Glutamine powder

2) Magnesium Citrate

3) Lactobacillus Sporogenes

Supplements for dysbiosis: see the chapter on dysbiosis.

Chapter 16:   PANCREAS (DIGESTIVE FUNCTION)

Anatomy and Physiology

The pancreas, besides producing insulin and glucagon, produces a number of substances that aid in our digestion of food. The glands producing these substances have ducts that enter the pancreatic duct, which then empties into the duodenum.

The digestive functions of the pancreas include the following:

1) Produces proteolytic (protein splitting) enzymes. These include: trypsin, chymotrypsin and carboxypolypeptidase which break down whole and partially digested proteins, and ribonuclease and deoxyribonuclease to split RNA and DNA.
2) Produces amylase to break down carbohydrates into disaccharides.
3) Produces lipase to break down neutral fat into fatty acids and glycerol.
4) Produces cholesterol esterase to hydrolyze cholesterol esters.
5) Secretes water and bicarbonate ions to make the pancreatic juice alkaline.

The digestive enzymes are secreted by the acinar cells of the pancreas, while it is the epithelial cells that secrete water and bicarbonate.

The chyme entering the small intestine is very acidic due to the HCl and pepsin from the stomach. The acidic chyme sends neural signals (via the vagus nerve) and hormonal signals (via secretin and cholecystokinin) to the pancreas causing large amounts of enzyme filled pancreatic juice to be released into the duodenum. The more acidic the chyme is, the more pancreatic juice is released to neutralize it. The alkaline juices prevent the stomach enzymes from eating through the duodenal wall and provide the perfect pH needed by the pancreatic enzymes. Any time the duodenal pH drops below 4.5, secretin is released, resulting in the release of bicarbonate.

Symptoms of Pancreatic (Digestive) Dysfunction

1) Gas and lower bowel discomfort, especially a few hours after a meal
2) A deficiency of bicarbonate can cause duodenal ulcers.
3) Fermentation, putrefaction and foul smelling stools are other possible symptoms

Causes of Pancreatic (Digestive) Dysfunction

1) Too many refined foods, too many combinations in one meal and eating between meals can all overwork the pancreas and eventually exhaust it.
2) Eating foods you are sensitive to will possibly cause the pancreas to over secrete enzymes in an attempt to break down the allergenic components and eventually deplete your enzyme supply.
3) Spinal misalignment in mid thoracic spine or cranial dysfunction irritating the vagus nerve can cause dysfunction.
4) A vitamin B deficiency from a bad diet or from eating refined products such as white sugar and white flour (they use up B vitamins in their digestion). Vitamin B is necessary for pancreatic enzyme production. These refined foods are also very acidic and thus over-stimulate the pancreas.
5) Hypochlorhydria will lead to less acidic chyme. This will cause decreased secretin output and thus decreased pancreatic output. Incomplete digestion may result. The primary cause, the hypochlorhydria in this case, needs correction in order for pancreatic function to be restored. (See the stomach chapter.)
6) Deficiency in the diet or poor assimilation of zinc (which is needed to form bicarbonate) can lead to sub-optimal bicarbonate formation. Zinc can be depleted by eating too many grains and other phytic acid containing foods. Mercury toxicity and eating foods you are sensitive to can also deplete zinc levels.
7) Taking sodium bicarbonate or other antacids can neutralize stomach contents and, as in #5, lead to decreased pancreatic output as a secondary condition.

Prevention and Treatment of Pancreatic (Digestive) Dysfunction

1) Avoid white sugar, white flour, white rice and other refined foods.
2) Don't eat in between meals and avoid too many food combinations

per meal.

3) Avoid foods you are sensitive to.

4) Eat foods high in B vitamins and zinc: whole grains, seeds, nuts, green vegetables and seaweed.

5) Avoid sodium bicarbonate and antacids. If you have gas, take a scoop of Takesumi Supreme to adsorb it.

6) If you suspect spinal misalignment or cranial dysfunction, see a good chiropractor.

7) Rub a reflex point on your left side between the 7th and 8th ribs where they meet the cartilage for 1 minute, 3 times a week, for 2 weeks.

8) Many people take digestive enzymes to help digestion. It is our opinion that, while this may bring symptomatic relief, it will not correct the underlying problem and may even suppress the pancreas from producing adequate enzymes. Also, many of the so called "vegetable enzymes" on the market are derived from fungi and we have found them to be highly allergenic, especially in patients who have had dysbiosis. Enzymes can be a temporary measure but try to correct the underlying problem.

9) Chew each mouthful thoroughly.

10) Eating raw pineapple and papaya at the beginning of a high protein meal can supply protein digesting enzymes and may prove helpful.

Supplement Recommendations

THORNE RESEARCH

1) DiPan9 - enzymes

Chapter 17:   **UTERUS**

Anatomy and Physiology

The uterus is located between the bladder and rectum in the pelvic cavity and weighs about 2 ounces. It is about the size of a pear and is made up of the following parts: the fundus (upper muscular portion above the entry of the fallopian tubes), the body (large central portion), isthmus (short narrowed portion between the body and cervix) and the cervix (narrow lower end which opens into the vagina).

Changing levels of estrogens and progesterone secreted by the corpus luteum promote secretory changes in the lining of the uterus (the endometrium) to prepare it for the implanting of a fertilized egg. At the time of ovulation, the cervix steps up mucus production to help the sperm get through to the egg. For the first twelve weeks after fertilization, the egg receives its nutrients from the large endometrial cells of the uterus.

Hormones, the menstrual cycle, and other factors involving the uterus, are discussed in the chapter on the ovaries to bring the interrelationship between FSH, LH, estrogen and progesterone together into one chapter. We suggest rereading the chapter on the ovaries at this time. It is beyond the scope of this book to discuss pregnancy and the anatomical and physiological changes accompanying it.

Symptoms of Uterine Dysfunction (others discussed in ovary chapter)

1) Prolonged or excessive bleeding during menses, leg aches prior to period, pelvic pain, and headaches at the very top of the head, can be possible signs of uterine dysfunction.

Causes of Uterine Dysfunction (others discussed in ovary chapter)

1) An I.U.D. can irritate the uterus and cause inflammation and bleeding in some cases.
2) Some causes of excessive uterine bleeding include: pituitary dysfunction causing excess estrogen, a congested liver not breaking

down excess estrogen, uterine polyps and ectopic pregnancy.

3) Spinal misalignment in the lumbar or sacral nerves can possibly cause uterine dysfunction.

4) Some risk factors for uterine cancer include: obesity, taking estrogen as hormone replacement without taking progesterone at the same time, never having been pregnant, and early onset of menses or late onset of menopause. All of these conditions can lead to increased or longer periods of estrogen exposure which can cause abnormal growth of the endometrial lining of the uterus.

5) Some indications for a hysterectomy (removal of uterus) include: uterine cancer, fibroids, endometriosis, uterine prolapse and excess bleeding.

6) As always, food sensitivities and dysbiosis may play a role.

Prevention and Treatment of Uterine Dysfunction

1) Eat a good diet low in sweets and refined fats. Have a qualified practitioner check you and your spouse or sexual partner for dysbiosis. (See the dysbiosis chapter.)

2) Rub a reflex point on the front of the pubic bone and also an area between the front and outside (antero-lateral) of both thighs, one minute daily for one week to aid in uterine problems.

3) Lie in the knee chest position for 60 seconds each night to prevent painful periods.

4) The following teas used internally have been reported helpful in correcting abnormal uterine discharge: lamb's quarters, huckleberry leaf and squaw vine.

5) Have a good chiropractor check for and correct spinal misalignment.

6) Apply a hot fomentation (107°) for 90 minutes daily, for 1 month, over the uterus and vagina to correct uterine inflammation.

7) Cold packs to either the breast, inner thigh, lumbar spine, or feet, will cause uterine contraction while hot packs will dilate uterine blood vessels and increase menstrual flow.

8) In some women, the uterus will drop out of position and can cause painful irregular periods and/or infertility. This often happens due to a weak levator ani or abdominal muscles or a distended colon. To treat this condition:

   a) Eat a high roughage diet and "fix" your colon. (See the large intestine chapter.)

b) Rub the reflex points mentioned in #2 and massage deeply over the abdominal and levator ani muscles, especially where the muscles attach to the bone.

c) Have a good chiropractor or someone knowledgeable in soft tissue manipulation perform a uterine lift technique. It is done externally and can have dramatic effects.

9) Jewish women have a lower rate of cervical cancer than other women. It is hypothesized that this is because Jewish women are more likely to marry Jewish men, and Jewish men are more likely to be circumcised.

Chapter 18: **PROSTATE**

Anatomy and Physiology

The prostate is a small gland encircling the urethra, about 1 1/2" wide, 1" thick, and 1" long, weighing about 1 ounce.

The prostate remains undeveloped throughout childhood and starts to grow at puberty due to the influence of testosterone, reaching full size and maturity at 20 years of age.

The prostate secretes a thin, milky, alkaline liquid that adds to the bulk of the semen. It helps neutralize the other acidic secretions composing the semen and raises the vaginal pH to a level that allows maximum sperm mobility and fertility. During ejaculation, the prostate, vas deferens, and seminal vesicles contract simultaneously.

Symptoms of Prostatic Dysfunction

1) The prostate can enlarge and become spongy (benign prostatic hypertrophy), exhibiting symptoms of difficult urination, incomplete urination, decreased force of urination, waking up a few times nightly to urinate, painful urination, dribbling after the flow stops and low back pain. If severe, urinary obstruction can occur.
2) Infection of the prostate (prostatitis) can have the above symptoms plus fever, chills and blood in urine.
3) Prostate cancer is the second leading cause of cancer related deaths in men. This cancer can also spread to the bones.

Causes of Prostate Dysfunction

1) Long term use of antihistamines can increase one's tendency toward, or aggravate cases of, benign prostatic hypertrophy.
2) Caffeine, poor nutritional assimilation (causing zinc and other deficiencies), bladder infections, more than one sexual partner and sexual excesses can cause prostate dysfunction.
3) Spinal misalignment in lumbar or sacral area can lead to prostate

issues.

4) Testes, pituitary or adrenal dysfunction can alter testosterone secretion and affect prostate development.
5) We have found that toxic metals, especially mercury, can lead to prostate problems. (See the toxic metal chapter.)
6) Dysbiosis can be a source of chronic prostate problems. (See the dysbiosis chapter.)
7) Eating foods you are sensitive to can cause prostate symptoms. (See the food sensitivity chapter.)

Prevention and Treatment of Prostate Dysfunction

1) Avoid taking antihistamines if possible and other drugs that may cause prostatic hypertrophy (do not stop any prescription medications before talking to your physician).
2) Rub a reflex point on the anterior pubic bone (one on each side), for 1 minute, every other day, for 2 weeks.
3) See a chiropractor to see if spinal misalignment is a contributing cause.
4) Abstain from alcohol, caffeine, tobacco, vinegar, and overly spicy foods.
5) Corn silk tea, garlic, kelp, burdock root and pumpkin seeds are all reported to be helpful in prostate problems.
6) Have a qualified practitioner check for food sensitivities, dysbiosis and toxic metal involvement. Your spouse or sexual partner needs to be checked as well because dysbiosis can be spread back and forth and needs to be eradicated in both for resolution. It is possible for the partner to be asymptomatic and still have the problem.
7) Walking strengthens the prostate.
8) A 110° enema or castor oil pack to the groin and inner thighs can be beneficial in prostate problems.
9) A hardened prostate will respond to sitting on a hot water bottle or to a hot footbath.
10) A cold sitz bath for 15 minutes can help relieve an inflamed prostate.
11) Eating foods high in plant sterols may relieve symptoms of prostate enlargement or prostate cancer. (See the ovary chapter.)

Recommended Products

THORNE RESEARCH

1) Basic Pygeum Herbal

2) Serenoa gelcaps

SUPREME NUTRITION PRODUCTS

3) Takesumi Supreme

Chapter 19: **SPLEEN**

Anatomy and Physiology

The spleen is a large organ in the lymphatic system working with the thymus, lymph and bone marrow. It is located in the left upper quadrant of the abdominal cavity, just below the diaphragm, behind the fundus of the stomach. It weighs between 5-7 ounces. It is vulnerable to being injured by fractures of the 9th, 10th and 11th ribs, and it is one of the few organs whose metabolic rate isn't controlled by the thyroid.

The spleen has the following functions:

1) Production/maturation of antibodies
2) Forms red blood cells in fetal life
3) Removes old and abnormal red blood cells, platelets and other damaged cells from circulation and reuses whatever parts it can
4) Filters out bacteria and parasites from the blood and lymph that have been killed by white blood cells
5) Acts as a reservoir for red blood cells and platelets that can be released when needed (blood loss, infection, hemorrhage, and strenuous exercise). These are released via signals of epinephrine from the adrenals and sympathetics.

It has been found that splenic tissue can sometimes regenerate after removal of the spleen. Howard Pearson at Yale University School of Medicine found that 13 of 22 children who had their spleens removed due to trauma had evidence of forming new splenic tissue within 1-8 years. It is hypothesized that a few old spleen cells left behind from the surgery triggered the regeneration.

Symptoms of Spleen Dysfunction

1) Symptoms of spleen dysfunction can include: paleness, anemia, tiredness, headaches, dizziness, irritability, left upper quadrant abdominal pain, a soapy taste in the mouth, nausea and being easily winded.

2) People with weak spleens are more prone to swollen glands, sore throat and infections. Their illnesses typically tend to last longer, often going on for weeks instead of days.

3) People with enlarged spleens get full easily due to its encroachment on the stomach. An enlarged spleen (splenomegaly) can be associated with illnesses such as lupus, mononucleosis and sickle cell disease.

Causes of Spleen Dysfunction

1) Anything that affects epinephrine release such as sugar, stress and hypoadrenia, can affect the spleen's ability to release blood cells and platelets. Taking epinephrine as a medication can also interfere.

2) Eating refined sugar can decrease the white blood cells' ability to travel to the sites where they are needed and engulf bacteria. An ice cream sundae contains about 24 teaspoons of sugar and can decrease white blood cell response by 92% for several hours after consumption.

3) Growth hormone is needed for proper spleen function. Anything interfering with the pituitary and growth hormone can also affect the spleen secondarily.

4) Spinal misalignment in the mid thoracics may affect spleen function.

Prevention and Treatment of Spleen Dysfunction

1) Make sure your thymus, adrenals, and pituitary are functioning correctly. (See their respective chapters.) If they are not, treat them.

2) Decrease your stress level and minimize your sugar intake.

3) Hot and cold showers beating down on your mid thoracic spine will stimulate the spleen.

4) Have a good chiropractor check for spinal misalignment.

5) Rub a reflex point located between the 7th and 8th ribs on the left side where they meet their cartilage. Do this for one minute, 3 times a week, for 1 month.

Recommended Supplements

THORNE RESEARCH

    1) Im-Encap

2) Myco-Immune

SUPREME NUTRITION PRODUCTS

3) Reishi Supreme

4) Thera Supreme

Chapter 20:   KIDNEYS

Anatomy and Physiology

The kidneys lie on the posterior abdominal wall, the left kidney being slightly higher than the right. They are fist sized, bean shaped, and weigh 5-6 ounces each. They each consist of an outer cortex containing glomeruli and tubules, and an inner medulla containing tubules. The 8-18 pyramids of the medulla open into calyces, which open into the renal pelvis, which will narrow into the ureter.

Approximately 1.2 liters of blood pass through the kidneys each minute and the kidneys contain about 70 miles of tubules.

The kidney cells are arranged in units called nephrons. Each nephron contains a glomerulus, Bowman's capsule, tubule and collecting duct. The glomerulus is a capillary network which blood enters through an afferent arteriole. Pressure forces fluid from the blood into Bowman's capsule (a funnel like structure), and from there into the tubules, and eventually the renal pelvis. The nephron (there are 1 million in each kidney) filters the blood, saving most of the water and important electrolytes. The rest: urea, creatinine, uric acid, excess sodium, potassium, chloride and hydrogen ions, are passed into the urine along with a few other substances the plasma secretes into the tubules. All in all, over 99% of the fluid is reabsorbed, as well as 99% of the sodium, 98% of the amino acids, almost 100% of the glucose, 88% of the potassium, 60% of the urea, etc. Antidiuretic hormone from the posterior pituitary and aldosterone from the adrenals influence urine volume and fluid retention.

The kidneys' main function is to control the volume, composition, and pressure of bodily fluids. Renin is a substance formed in the juxtaglomerular apparatus of the kidneys. It acts as a catalyst in forming angiotensin. Angiotensin stimulates aldosterone secretion by the adrenals. This mechanism affects our blood pressure. Angiotensin causes the kidneys' efferent arterioles to constrict. This constriction increases renal tubular reabsorption, thus increasing blood volume and pressure. Atrial Natriuretic Factor, released from the heart, is an antagonistic hormone to angiotensin, resulting in the overall effect of lowering blood volume and pressure.

Symptoms of Kidney Dysfunction

1) Symptoms of kidney dysfunction can include fatigue, weight loss, edema, flank pain, abnormal blood pressure, nausea, a bad taste in the mouth, blurred vision, acidosis and a puffy face.
2) In kidney dysfunction, urine output can be decreased or increased. The urine can be cloudy or contain blood, and you may wake up several times nightly to urinate.
3) Chills and fever often accompany kidney infections.
4) Kidney stone symptoms can include pain (very severe at times), loss of appetite, nausea, vomiting, paleness, sweating, chills, fever and blood in urine.

Causes of Kidney Dysfunction

1) Birth control pills, many other medications (including diuretics), a high intake of sugar and/or meat, not drinking enough water and EDTA (a food additive, also used in chelation therapy) can all cause kidney damage.
2) The protein in cows' milk, and also refined sugar, can stimulate kidney stone formation.
3) Parathyroid dysfunction, due to its effects on calcium and phosphate absorption, can lead to secondary kidney dysfunction.
4) Hypoadrenia (see the adrenal chapter) can cause the adrenals not to respond to angiotensin and cause resultant blood pressure problems.
5) Spinal misalignment in the lower thoracic spine can cause kidney dysfunction.
6) A diet too high in protein can cause kidney hypertrophy, due to the extra work the kidney must perform to rid the body of excess nitrogen and protein byproducts. Over time, this can cause kidney dysfunction. Excess protein intake will also cause the body to excrete more calcium; this can cause kidney stones and/or osteoporosis.
7) Trauma or loss of muscle tone can cause the kidney to drop down (ptosis). This can cause a kink in the ureter and decrease urinary output. Someone trained in soft tissue manipulation can check for this.
8) High blood pressure or exposure to cold without dressing warmly

enough can cause increased urine output and overwork the kidneys.

9) Alcohol retards pituitary ADH output, as does caffeine. This would cause an increase in urine output.

10) Nicotine stimulates ADH production leading to decreased urine output.

11) Other pituitary dysfunction can cause altered ADH output and influence the kidneys.

12) The methylxanthine family (coffee, tea, chocolate, etc.) can irritate the kidneys as can eating foods you are sensitive to, dysbiosis and toxic metals/chemicals. (See their respective chapters.)

Prevention and Treatment of Kidney Dysfunction

1) Drink at least 6-8 glasses of water daily and minimize salt intake. Don't eat too much protein. Don't take refined protein powder supplements unless you are certain you have a protein deficiency.

2) Avoid foods high in oxalic acid such as spinach, rhubarb, chocolate and chard. Don't overdose on calcium supplements.

3) Don't smoke.

4) Alcohol, white sugar, white flour, milk, birth control pills and lack of exercise can all be damaging to the kidneys and increase susceptibility to kidney stone formation.

5) High blood pressure can be due to bad kidneys, adrenals, thyroid, diet, cranial dysfunction, etc. Find the cause.

6) The following herbs may be beneficial in kidney problems: burdock root, chaparral, kidney bean pod, corn silk, wild Oregon grape, chamomile, cleavers, milkweed, thistle, nettle, sorrel and uva ursi.

7) The following foods may benefit the kidneys: parsley, watercress, melon, cucumber, garlic, banana and honey (in small amounts).

8) If you suspect spinal misalignment, food sensitivity, dysbiosis, or toxic metals (see their respective chapters), see a qualified natural health care practitioner.

9) Rub 2 reflex points: each is one inch above and one inch to the side of the umbilicus. Rub them for 1 minute each, 3 times a week, for 1 month.

10) For calcium oxalate stones, acidify the genitourinary tract using cranberry juice. If the stones are uric acid, alkalinize the body using plantain tea, fresh grapefruit juice and lots of raw vegetables and fruits (except cranberries and plums).

11) A cold footbath aids in bladder and kidney bleeding.

12) A mud bath to the whole body (except the head) is helpful in removing wastes and takes a load off overworked kidneys.

One dramatic case involved a friend of ours. One Saturday morning many years ago, he had his third attack of kidney stones. Previous attacks put him in the hospital for a week at a time with excruciating pain, vomiting, etc. At those times he was on extensive pain medication orally and intravenously.

In this episode, we determined through history and urine pH that it was probably a uric acid stone. A group of 20 friends got together and prayed. We put a large hot fomentation over his lower thoracics and lumbar spine and folded it over onto his abdomen. We had him drink lots of plantain tea and fresh grapefruit juice. Within 3-4 hours his symptoms were totally gone. The hot fomentations dilated the ureter and allowed the stone to pass. Please try this only under a doctor's supervision.

Recommended Products

SUPREME NUTRITION PRODUCTS

1) Body Guard Supreme is an herb that has been used traditionally for centuries in cases with kidney and gall stones. As with any regimen, consult your physician.

Find the cause (foods, dysbiosis, metals, etc) and look in those chapters for products.

Chapter 21:   BLADDER

Anatomy and Physiology

The bladder is a sac-like organ in the pelvis, located just above and behind the pubic bone, which stores the urine produced by the kidneys. The bladder is composed of 4 layers: epithelium (lines the bladder and is in contact with the urine), lamina propria (under the epithelium; a layer of connective tissue and blood vessels), detrusor muscle (also called muscularis propria; the main muscle layer of the bladder made of thick smooth muscle that forms the bladder wall) and perivesical soft tissue (outermost layer of fat, fibrous tissue and blood vessels). The bladder has a capacity of up to about 24 ounces. There are two tubular structures called ureters (one from each kidney) that drain urine into the bladder. The urethra acts as an outflow tract and takes urine from the bladder to the exterior for elimination. The internal urethral sphincter is the muscle at the junction of the urinary bladder and the urethra. It is this muscle that keeps the opening to the urethra closed until there is enough urine in the bladder to stretch the walls and initiate a neurological reflex, causing the bladder to contract and the internal urethral sphincter to relax. Even after the reflex occurs, the brain can keep the external sphincter closed and prevent urination.

Symptoms of Bladder Dysfunction

1) Symptoms of bladder dysfunction can include burning and frequent urination, cloudy urine with pus and/or blood and low back or abdominal pain.
2) With bladder infection, fever and chills are also common symptoms. Women's urethras are only 1-2" long, while men's are 8-12" long. This is one reason women are more prone to bladder infections (bacteria from the outside can reach a woman's bladder more easily).

Causes of Bladder Dysfunction

1) Dysbiosis can be a major cause of bladder infections. Be sure to have your spouse or sexual partner checked as well.

2) Overly spicy food, mustard, pepper, alcohol, birth control pills, caffeine and foods high in oxalic acid (spinach, rhubarb, and chocolate) make you more prone to getting bladder infections.

3) Eating foods you're sensitive to, especially milk, can increase your likelihood of getting a bladder infection or an irritable bladder.

4) Spinal alignment in the lumbar or sacral nerves can decrease your resistance (as can a weak immune system) and cause bladder problems.

5) An imbalance in the abdominal muscles with painful nodules upon palpating; these muscles can cause pain in the bladder with associated sphincter spasm and residual urine.

6) Too much refined starch and sugar can irritate the bladder.

7) Aniline dyes and tobacco tars are suspected of causing bladder cancer.

8) It has been our experience that toxic metal and chemical exposure can irritate the bladder, leading to frequent but low volume urinations.

Prevention and Treatment of Bladder Dysfunction

1) Correct dysbiosis. (See the dysbiosis chapter.)

2) Avoid alcohol, sugar, caffeine, foods high in oxalic acid, overly spicy foods, birth control pills, tampons, feminine deodorant sprays and spermicides.

3) Avoid foods you're sensitive to.

4) For bladder infections: eat lots of watermelon and pumpkin seeds, drink 1 cup of buchu tea per hour and eat several raw cloves of garlic daily for 5 days. Take a hot sitz bath twice daily. If your urine pH is over seven, drink unsweetened cranberry juice and take ascorbic acid to acidify the urine. If urine pH is 5.5 or lower, eat mainly fruits and vegetables (minimal grains and meats) to make the urine more basic and try taking D-Mannose (the active component in cranberry juice, but as an isolated supplement, should not acidify an already acidic urine). The goal in treating these types of infections is often to shift the pH to one that is unfriendly to the infecting organism.

5) If you suspect spinal or sacral misalignment, see a good chiropractor.

6) Cleavers, wasabi, golden seal, slippery elm, wild carrot and chamomile may also be healing to the bladder.

7) Check for tender nodules in your abdominal muscles. If you find a nodule, bend backwards and put pressure with your thumb on the

nodule until the tenderness subsides. Do this to all the nodules you find.

8) For women, the following may help: when going to the bathroom, wipe from front to back to prevent bacteria from entering your urethra, take showers instead of baths, cleanse your genital area before and after sexual intercourse, avoid using feminine hygiene sprays and use only white unscented toilet paper to avoid potential dye reactions.

9) Children who wet their beds often have food sensitivities. Eliminating the food sensitivity and rubbing the points in #10 often eliminates the problem.

10) Rub the anterior pubic bone on each side for 1 minute daily for 1 week to stimulate bladder cleansing.

11) Drink lots of water and wear only cotton or silk underwear.

Recommended Supplements

THORNE RESEARCH

1) Uristatin

2) Ascorbic Acid

Dysbiosis correcting supplements; see the dysbiosis chapter.

Michael Lebowitz DC and Ami Kapadia MD

Chapter 22:   **HEART**

Anatomy and Physiology

The heart is the muscular pump of the circulatory system. It is surrounded by a sac known as the pericardium. The heart has 4 chambers; right and left atrium, right and left ventricle. It weighs about 12 ounces, is 6 inches long, 4 inches wide, beats 2 1/2 billion times in the average lifetime, and pumps 7000 quarts of blood daily through 60,000 miles of blood vessels. The heart rests 1/2 second between beats. Even though it is only 1/200th of the body's weight, it uses 1/20th of the blood supply. At rest, the heart pumps 4-5 liters per minute, this can increase to 20-30 liters during heavy exercise.

Deoxygenated blood from the body enters the heart through the right atrium, goes through the tricuspid valve to the right ventricle, through the pulmonary semilunar valve (also known as the pulmonic valve) and is pumped to the lungs. There, it picks up oxygen and goes to the left atrium, through the mitral valve to the left ventricle, and through the aortic semilunar valve (also known as the aortic valve) to the rest of the body.

Contraction of the atrium helps pump blood into the ventricles, though about 70% of the blood goes in before contraction takes place. With ventricular contraction, the A-V valves (tricuspid and mitral) are closed to prevent backflow into the atria. During this time, blood collects in the atrium. Ventricular contraction also causes the semilunar (aortic and pulmonic) valves to be pushed open for blood to leave the heart. As blood enters the large arteries, the pressure builds up and shuts the semilunar valves. The blood buildup in the atria then forces the A-V valves open and the cycle repeats.

When listening with a stethoscope, the low-pitched sound (or first heart sound) is caused by blood bouncing off the A-V valves after closing to prevent backflow from the ventricles, while the rapid snap of the second sound is that blood bouncing off of the aortic and pulmonic valves after closing to prevent backflow from the arteries to the ventricles.

The normal heart beats about 72 times per minute. Intense parasympathetic stimulation can decrease it to 20-30 beats per minute. Intense sympathetic stimulation can increase the heart rate to 250-300 beats per minute.

The S-A node in the right atrium controls the heart rate by generating action potentials at the rate of about 100 beats per minute (bpm), which at rest is lowered to approximately 72 bpm from acetylcholine release onto the S-A node from the vagus nerve. The S-A node fibers go into the atrium causing it to contract. The fibers also stimulate the A-V node which delays the impulse about 1/10th of a second before it travels through the Purkinje fibers to cause the ventricles to contract.

Parasympathetic and sympathetic fibers attach to the S-A and A-V nodes to change the heart rate when necessary. Pressure on the spinal nerves from the upper thoracic spine can irritate the sympathetic fibers and affect the heart rate.

Heavy exercise over many weeks and months will cause the heart muscle to hypertrophy and the chambers of the ventricles to enlarge. This increases the effectiveness of the heart by allowing it to pump more blood with each beat, thus less beats are needed.

Heavy exercise will also cause more blood vessels ("collaterals") to the heart to be built to increase its food supply. This will also decrease the likelihood of heart attack. The arteries supplying the heart are known as the coronary arteries.

Symptoms of Heart Dysfunction

By the age of 16-20 years, over 1/2 the population shows evidence of hardening of the arteries. Symptoms of heart dysfunction can include:

1) Irregular heart beat
2) Pain in the chest that may travel down the left arm
3) Fatigue with exertion
4) Being easily winded
5) Coughing frequently, restlessness, pallor
6) Increased anxiety

7) Swelling in the lower legs
8) Angina is a pressure or squeezing sensation especially in the mid or upper sternal region on the left side. It can radiate to the neck, jaw, and teeth, and can increase during exercise.

Causes of Heart Dysfunction

In the U.S., there are close to 1 million deaths per year due to cardiovascular disease. It is estimated that over 10 million Americans suffer from this disease. Causes of cardiovascular disease:

1) Smoking increases the risk of heart disease. Female smokers are nine times more likely to die from coronary heart disease than non-smokers. Deaths in general from coronary heart disease are 70% higher in smokers.
2) Consuming caffeine and other methylxanthines in excess can lead to heartbeat irregularities in susceptible individuals.
3) A diet high in sugar is detrimental to heart health. Diets high in refined carbohydrates (white sugar, white flour, etc.) can cause the liver to over manufacture cholesterol.
4) Birth control pills and estrogen replacement therapy may increase the likelihood of heart problems.
5) A diet too high in protein increases cardiac output by 30% to aid digestion. This, if done habitually, can overwork the heart.
6) A toxic bowel won't be able to eliminate cholesterol well and can lead to fatty deposits in the blood vessels.
7) A person with an under active thyroid will have an increased amount of fat in the blood and be more susceptible to elevated cholesterol levels. (See the thyroid chapter.)
8) Hypoadrenia, causing lowered aldosterone output, can cause electrolyte imbalances and resultant heartbeat abnormalities, as can ileocecal valve syndrome (see their respective chapters).
9) Spinal misalignment in the upper thoracic spine as well as rib subluxations may cause heart problems.
10) A vitamin B deficiency can cause heart palpitations.
11) Ulcer patients fed a high milk diet have twice the incidence of heart attacks as ulcer patients not on a high milk diet.
12) Vegetarian Seventh-day Adventists suffer from 84% less coronary heart disease than the general population (most abstain from tobacco, caffeine, alcohol, and meat). Non-vegetarian Seventh-day

Adventists suffer from 45% less coronary heart disease.

13) A lack of magnesium appears to produce heart problems. Low hydrochloric acid, a high protein diet, too high an intake of dairy products and a diet high in refined foods all tend to produce magnesium deficiencies.

14) Fat in the blood damages arterial walls and causes hardening of the arteries. Diets high in trans fats tend to create this change. Trans fats include anything listed as "partially hydrogenated fat." These trans fats can be found in margarine, pre-made baked goods, many foods prepared in restaurants, etc.

15) Alcohol and trans fats can be pro-inflammatory and may cause red blood cells to clump together. This can block blood flow to capillaries causing decreased oxygen supply and damage to the circulatory system and the cells it supplies nutrients to.

16) Hardening of the arteries due to any of the above causes or any other factor that decreases oxygen supply can cause angina.

17) A hiatal hernia can mimic heart problems. (See the stomach chapter.)

18) A hypertonic nodule on the right pectoralis major muscle between the 5th and 6th ribs may cause increased heart rate and premature contractions. Deactivating the nodule by deep manual pressure for 2 minutes will cause the symptoms to cease. A hypertonic nodule on the left pectoralis major can cause pain radiation down the left arm mimicking heart problems. When deactivating these, palpate for the exact location (it should initially be quite tender and aggravate the symptoms with pressure) and put sustained pressure on it while the muscle is in a stretched position.

19) Deficiencies of the amino acid carnitine, coenzyme-Q10 and essential fatty acids, can all have negative consequences on the heart.

Prevention and Treatment of Heart Dysfunction

1) Abstain from tobacco, caffeine, grain-fed meat, trans fats and sugar.

2) Don't overeat in general and don't eat too much protein, sugar or fat. Get your weight down to a normal level. For every 5 pounds of extra weight you carry, your body needs 4 more miles of blood vessels.

3) Minimize salt intake to help maintain blood pressure. Deficiencies of magnesium, potassium and/or calcium can also lead to hypertension in some individuals.

4) Sunlight can cause cholesterol on the skin to change to vitamin D. As

you get more and more sunlight, the body will bring more cholesterol to the surface. A two-hour sunbath can lower serum cholesterol levels by 13%. Sunlight can also lower blood pressure between 6-40mm and this drop will last 5-6 days. Pulse rate will also decrease.

5) Make sure your thyroid, adrenals, liver and colon are all working correctly and not causing heart dysfunction.

6) Exercise will strengthen the heart muscle, allowing each beat to pump more blood. Less beats are needed and the heart will get the "rest" it needs. Exercise will decrease your resting pulse and blood pressure. Exercise will also build up your collateral circulation, growing more blood vessels to the heart to supply it with oxygen and nutrients. This decreases the likelihood of coronary heart disease.

7) In people with a family history of heart attacks, consider taking an L-carnitine supplement to strengthen the heart. Coenzyme-Q10 and essential fatty acids can also help. For meat eaters, grass fed meat can supply all of these factors if eaten regularly.

Recommended Products

THORNE RESEARCH

1) L-Carnitine

2) Omega3 with CoQ10

3) Super EPA

4) Perfusia

5) Cal-Mag Citrate Powder

6) Magnesium Citramate

7) Potassium Citrate

Michael Lebowitz DC and Ami Kapadia MD

Chapter 23:   LUNGS

Anatomy and Physiology

The lungs are the main organs of our respiratory system. The right lung is composed of 3 lobes and weighs a little over a pound. The left lung weighs a little under a pound and consists of 2 lobes. The trachea enters the lungs and branches out into bronchi, and then bronchioles (about .01 inches in diameter), and eventually into 250 million air sacs called alveoli. Capillaries bring blood low in oxygen and high in carbon dioxide to the lungs. The carbon dioxide diffuses into the alveoli for removal and oxygen is transferred to the capillaries.

We normally have a respiration rate of approximately 12-16 breaths per minute (a range of 12-20 is considered normal), inhaling about 1 pint with each inspiration. The lungs hold about 1 gallon of air. During sleep we require about 2 gallons of air per minute and this can increase by 600% during exercise. During heavy exercise we need up to twenty times as much oxygen as during resting.

The lungs are somewhat elastic and expand and contract during breathing. The contraction and expansion of the diaphragm, elevation and depression of the ribs, and actions of the abdominal muscles, scalenes and quadratus lumborum, all play a role. During inhalation, the diaphragm moves downward and the lungs expand. This causes the pressure in the lungs to decrease and air flows in. During exhalation, the diaphragm moves up, the lungs contract, the pressure in the lungs increases and air flows out.

Cilia are located along the air passages to and in the lungs. They help trap particles and they beat toward the pharynx to remove the particles and excessive mucus.

The lungs normally contain about 1 pint of blood but they can act as a blood reservoir carrying up to 3 pints (to release the extra when needed).

Symptoms of Lung Dysfunction

1) Symptoms of bronchitis include muscle pain, sore throat, coughing, wheezing and respiratory tract infection.
2) Symptoms of asthma include difficulty breathing, wheezing, shortness of breath, tightness, coughing and increased heart rate.
3) In emphysema, the alveoli become distended and rupture due to irritation. Carbon dioxide becomes trapped in the lungs and exhalation is difficult. There is a decreased number of pulmonary capillaries and a decreased capacity of the lungs to oxygenate the blood. Shortness of breath and lack of energy are common symptoms.
4) Symptoms of lung cancer include coughing, wheezing, chest pain, weakness, weight loss and expelling blood from the lungs.

Causes of Lung Dysfunction

1) Smoking is the most common cause of lung problems. People who habitually smoke more than two packs of cigarettes daily are 20-30 times as likely to develop lung cancer as non-smokers. Women smoking at least 10 cigarettes daily are 7.4 times as likely to die of lung cancer as non-smokers. Parents who smoke increase a child's risk of developing lung problems. Bronchitis and asthma are also aggravated by smoking (90% of all people suffering from bronchitis are smokers).
2) Besides smoking, hypoadrenia, eating dairy products if you are sensitive to them, gas heat, and wood stoves can all contribute to or cause bronchitis.
3) Asbestos, uranium ore and nickel dust can also cause lung cancer.
4) Asthma has many causes. Most asthmatics suffer from fungal problems. (See the dysbiosis chapter.) This can easily be contracted by breathing in molds or even sexual transmission. Aspirin, emotional trauma, molds, allergies (especially dairy), growing up on artificial infant formula, sodium bisulphate (used in salad bars to keep lettuce from wilting), sulphur dioxide (in car exhaust and used to preserve dried fruit), sodium benzoate (a common food preservative) and animal dander can all trigger asthma attacks.
5) Living in the city or near other sources of air pollution can cause most types of lung diseases.
6) Spinal misalignment in the upper thoracic area can cause lung

problems.

7) Paraquat is an herbicide that was previously used on millions of acres of farmland in the U.S. It made tilling unnecessary before planting soybeans, wheat, corn, sunflowers and cotton. In Hawaii, it was used to kill dogs and also on some crops. It has been detected in some towns' water supplies. Paraquat is extremely dangerous and often fatal. It concentrates in the lungs, makes them red, soft, and brittle and increases their weight by 150%. The lungs become filled with fibrous tissue, oxygen passage is blocked and you slowly suffocate. It is most often lethal. In minute doses blood clots and decreased oxygen passage are the main effects. Paraquat has been banned for most uses, but still may contaminate water supplies, crops, etc. One study found the half life of paraquat varied from 16 months to 13 years. Clay taken soon after the exposure is the only known antidote.

Prevention and Treatment of Lung Dysfunction

1) Don't smoke. Avoid living in an area with heavy air pollution.
2) Heavy exercise and abdominal breathing help clear the lungs. Sunlight speeds up the removal of dust and particles from the lungs.
3) Borage tea and slippery elm tea may be helpful in lung conditions, as is a mixture of lemon juice and fig juice (from soaking dried figs overnight).
4) Antihistamines dry up secretions and make particulates harder to expel in lung problems. They should be avoided if possible.
5) If you suspect spinal misalignment as a possible cause, see a good chiropractor.
6) Rub 2 reflex points between the 3rd and 4th ribs next to the sternum, 1 minute daily, for 2 weeks, to stimulate the lungs.
7) For emphysema - stop smoking, get lots of exercise, and eat garlic and lots of raw fruits and vegetables.
8) For bronchitis - stop smoking, check your adrenals, and eliminate dairy products. The following herbs are reported helpful as teas: mullein, milkweed, coltsfoot, chickweed, and anise. A poultice of charcoal and flaxseed or onion is reported helpful, as is hot and cold fomentations (to the chest) or showers (3 minutes hot followed by 30 seconds cold).
9) For asthma:

    a) Find the cause. Check for fungal problems and get rid of mold in the home and work environment. (See the dysbiosis chapter.) Evaluate the adrenals, pancreas, thyroid, pituitary, liver, thymus, and spleen.

b) Stay on the adrenal recovery diet for 2-3 months and then, afterwards, only allow a minimum amount of sweets (2 tablespoons per week in all your foods is the maximum allowed). No dairy, alcohol, marijuana, tobacco or unnecessary medications (do not stop any medications without the consent of your physician). Stay off all foods you are sensitive to. Get rid of indoor pets and stay away from animals if necessary.

c) Go out to the forest and seashore as often as possible. Air charged with positive ions in artificially heated or air conditioned buildings can aggravate asthma. Sunlight is very beneficial for asthmatics.

d) Develop a good posture, dress warmly, and give yourself a dry brush massage daily (a loofah sponge is ideal) to increase elimination.

e) Breathe deeply. About once every hour forcefully expel all your air.

f) Keep your home dust and mold free and avoid second hand smoke.

10) During acute asthma attacks:

a) Depress the soft spot behind the angle of your jaw (on each side) for 2 minutes. Also press in beneath the sternoclavicular joint for 2 minutes. These will inhibit vagus and phrenic nerve function and often calm acute attacks.

b) Hot packs on the chest or pouring cold water on the back of the neck for 90 seconds are reported to relieve acute attacks.

c) Drinking 2 cloves of garlic blended in hot water may help alleviate an attack, as may passion flower tea and inhaling eucalyptus.

d) Forcefully expelling all your air through a small straw into a gallon of water can help relieve an acute attack.

e) Magnesium and/or molybdenum supplementation can often help.

f) Call your physician.

We have also found that, as a general rule for both allergies and asthma, the longer a patient has been on steroidal medication to control the condition, the longer it takes for his/her body to heal. It appears that the medication brings short-term relief but weakens the body and creates a long-term problem. Steroids also make it much harder to correct fungal dysbiosis. However, you should never go off prescribed asthma or allergy medication without the help of a licensed physician.

Recommended Supplements

THORNE RESEARCH

1) T Asmatica Plus

2) Magnesium Citramate

3) Molybdenum Picolinate

Supplements to correct dysbiosis; see the chapter on dysbiosis.

PART 2:   ROOT CAUSES OF ILLNESS

The next several chapters will address what we feel are common root causes of illness and will be based primarily on clinical experience with some reference to background information to help in overall understanding. We will be covering the following major contributors to illness: dysbiosis (with reference to specific pathogens), heavy metals, food allergies/toxins and neurotransmitter imbalances. While we will often list typical symptoms associated with a certain bug/toxin/food allergy, it is useful to keep in mind a key point often recited by the founder of Applied Kinesiology, Dr. George Goodheart D.C., who said that "anything can cause anything." For example, it is possible for the same trigger to cause fatigue in one patient but cause migraines in another. It is also possible for multiple different triggers to cause a specific symptom. There is no way to predict which trigger will cause which symptom in a patient. Often, different triggers can produce overlapping symptoms, so that there is no direct correlation between each specific trigger and each specific symptom. Also, a specific trigger might not cause the same symptom each time. Thus, the overall goal in relieving symptomatology and achieving health is to find as many imbalances (bugs, toxins, food allergies, etc.) as possible and correct them in an effort to achieve the best overall outcome for each person.

While a patient may recall his/her illness beginning after a specific exposure/event, that exposure/event is often the final "straw that broke the camel's back" rather than the ultimate cause of the illness. It is more often the "total load" or the combination of many different factors that results in illness, rather than an isolated infection, toxin, etc. It is important to keep the total load concept in mind as you begin to unravel the causes of illness.

While we will be discussing specific treatment recommendations for each root cause, it is always important to follow general health-promoting lifestyle practices. These include the following:

1) Spending as much time in the natural outdoors as possible with appropriate sunlight exposure

2) Getting at least 7-8 hours of sleep regularly and going to sleep by 10:00 pm
3) Living as naturally as possible by avoiding chemicals in cleaning products and personal care products
4) Taking steps to reduce stress
5) Eating a nutrient-dense diet that is low in processed foods and sugar
6) Eating bacterially cultured raw foods when possible such as sauerkraut, kefir, yogurt, etc. assuming you are not sensitive to those foods
7) Avoiding foods you are sensitive to/intolerant of, and limiting alcohol intake. Both of these steps will help you to maintain a healthy intestinal lining.

All of the above steps will help to create a robust immune system that can better resist illness and disease.

Chapter 24:   **DYSBIOSIS/MICROBES**

The first root cause of illness we will be discussing is related to "dysbiosis." Dysbiosis is defined as a state of altered microbial ecology that causes or contributes to disease/dysfunction. Organisms of low intrinsic virulence, such as bacteria, yeast and protozoa/parasites, induce disease or dysfunction by altering the nutrition, neuroendocrine and/or immunologic responses of a person. In other words, there are billions of organisms that reside in each of us as part of our normal flora. These organisms are vitally important to the development and maintenance of a healthy immune system. Just a few of their critical functions involve: warding off pathogens, decreasing allergic responses, and helping in the excretion of toxins. When this natural microbial balance is disrupted, illness can result. Our goal in treating dysbiosis is to eliminate pathogens, which in turn, will help to normalize mucosal function and immunity. Below, we will discuss the different organisms/pathogens that can be involved in dysbiosis. For each category of pathogens, we will discuss sources of infection, symptoms that can be related and prevention/treatment.

PARASITES

A parasite is a living organism that subsists at the expense of its host. A parasite can cause a variety of symptoms as your immune system reacts to its unwelcome presence. In this group, we are including worms and single-celled organisms that may be found in the stool, as well as parasites that can exist in other body systems besides the gastrointestinal tract.

Sources

1) Water/food contamination (more common when eating out vs. cooking at home)
2) Overseas exposure/travel
3) Sexual partners (exchange of saliva can be enough to spread infection)

4) Pets

Most common symptoms

1) Abdominal pain, nausea/vomiting, constipation/diarrhea
2) Irritable bowel syndrome
3) Skin rashes, eczema
4) Chronic pain
5) Fibromyalgia syndrome (FMS), chronic fatigue syndrome (CFS)
6) Nutrient depletion
7) Night sweats/chills
8) Abnormal weight loss

Prevention.

1) Filter water
2) Be as careful as possible with food sources and restaurant choices .
3) Have your partner checked to avoid infection/re-infection.
4) Don't let pets lick your face and wash your hands often if you have a lot of contact with animals.

Supplement Recommendations

SUPREME NUTRITION PRODUCTS

1) Morinda Supreme

2) Melia Supreme

3) Golden Thread Supreme

4) Oral Defense

THORNE RESEARCH

5) Artecin

6) Berbercap

7) Juglans Nigra

It is optimal to work in conjunction with a well versed alternative medicine physician when treating dysbiosis.

FUNGI

Yeast species are a normal part of our gastrointestinal ecology. However, problems arise when the yeasts overgrow and cause symptoms through a variety of mechanisms. Many aspects of modern day living favor the overgrowth of yeast, from pharmaceuticals to poor diet to environmental exposures, which will be discussed below.

While practitioners and patients involved in alternative/holistic medicine have been aware of "candida" related problems for the last few decades, there are many other species of fungi/yeast besides candida albicans that can be problematic. We do not distinguish between candida overgrowth/infections and other fungal infections because the treatment we recommend is the same regardless of the species you have. As we will discuss in the causes of fungal infections below, there are sources of exposure that you may not know about. It is important to avoid all sources in order to prevent recurrent symptoms from fungus.

Causes

1) Antibiotics
2) Steroid use (prednisone, etc.), including steroid inhalers
3) Birth control pills/hormone replacement therapy may contribute to the problem, but may not be enough to cause the problem on their own. This is less common with bio-identical hormones compared to synthetic hormones.
4) Mold exposure (via inhalation or skin contact) through workplace, home, etc.
5) Hot, humid environments (contribute to mold formation/exposure)
6) Sexual partner (exchange of saliva can be enough to spread infection)

7) Pets

Common Symptoms

1) Fatigue
2) Brain fog
3) Abdominal symptoms, nausea/vomiting, constipation/diarrhea, bloating/flatulence
4) GERD (reflux)
5) Depression, mood swings, and other psychiatric conditions
6) Migraines/headaches
7) Difficulty concentrating
8) Skin rashes, eczema, psoriasis
9) Asthma, respiratory problems
10) Nutrient depletion
11) Chronic pain
12) FMS/CFS
13) Recurrent subluxations
14) Arthritis
15) ADHD (can also contribute to autism spectrum disorders)
16) Thrush, vaginal yeast infection
17) Inability to lose weight
18) Chemical sensitivities

Prevention

1) Avoid antibiotics, prednisone, and hormones unless absolutely necessary (do not stop any prescription medications without consulting a physician). If prescription antibiotics are necessary, follow measures to prevent overgrowth of yeasts (i.e. consider taking Morinda Supreme at the same time as the medication and follow up with probiotics, eating cultured foods, and possibly taking one of the antimicrobials listed below under treatment).
2) Avoid mold exposure in work/home environment. Dehumidification may be necessary in hot/humid climates. Diffusing essential oils such as cedar oil and tea tree oil can help to lower indoor mold counts. Washing floors and walls with a borax/water solution or tea tree oil/water solution can also greatly help to reduce mold counts. If you find a water leak or water damage, and there is a possibility of mold growth, it is essential to fix the problem as soon as possible. After it is

fixed, the above measures such as the essential oils and borax solution can be used. An ozonator can also be used after an area of water damage is fixed to further ensure eradication of mold. However, caution must be used when using an ozonator. We recommend you discuss its use with a practitioner knowledgeable in environmental medicine and stay out of the house while ozonating.

3) Have your partner checked to avoid infection/re-infection.

Supplement Recommendations

SUPREME NUTRITION PRODUCTS

1) Morinda Supreme

2) Melia Supreme

3) Golden Thread Supreme

4) Oral Defense

THORNE RESEARCH

5) SF-722

6) Undecyn

Strictly adhering to a special diet during the 2-3 weeks of treatment for yeast/fungus is essential. You must avoid any foods with sweetening (sugar, honey, maple syrup, corn syrup, barley malt, etc.), fruit juice, dried fruit, vinegar, alcohol, soy sauce, miso, cheese, and yeast. Stevia, freshly made vegetable juice (if less than 50% carrot), unsweetened grapefruit juice and unsweetened lemon juice along with all fresh fruit are OK. You should also be checked for food sensitivities/food toxins, and avoid all that you are found to be sensitive to during the treatment period. We check for these through Applied Kinesiology testing, but there are other methods that can be used. If you do not have access to a practitioner that can check for you, it is best to avoid the major food toxins during treatment: gluten, dairy, corn, egg, soy, and solanines.

It is very helpful to have your sexual partner tested (or simply treated) as well or recidivism is possible through re-infection if he/she is a fungal carrier. If the fungus problem is not resolved within a few weeks it is most often due to a hidden fungal/mold problem in the house or your sexual partner being a carrier. If these are not addressed the problem can persist indefinitely.

VIRUS

When we think of viruses, most of us think of colds and respiratory infections. However, there are many different types of viruses that can cause a wide range of symptoms, as will be discussed below. Symptoms from a virus can last anywhere from a few days to indefinitely.

Causes

1) Airborne
2) Sexual partner (exchange of saliva can be enough to pass infection)
3) Pets

Common Symptoms

1) Respiratory symptoms (rhinitis/sinusitis, pneumonia, cough, sore throat, etc)
2) Abdominal pain, nausea/vomiting, constipation/diarrhea
3) Headaches
4) Fatigue
5) Night sweats/chills
6) FMS/CFS
7) Skin rashes
8) Swollen glands, especially cervical

Prevention

1) General hygiene practices (wash hands before eating, etc.)
2) If you work in a hospital/doctor's office where you are around sick people, air purifiers can be used to decrease airborne transmission.

3) Have your partner checked to avoid infection/re-infection.

4) Eat a low sugar (or better yet, no refined sugar) diet.

Supplement Recommendations

SUPREME NUTRITION PRODUCTS

1) Morinda Supreme

2) Melia Supreme

3) Golden Thread Supreme

4) Oral Defense

5) Thera Supreme

6) Reishi Supreme

7) Camu Supreme

THORNE RESEARCH

8) Isatis

9) IM Encap

10) Arabinex

11) Vitamin C with Flavanoids

12) Olive Leaf Extract

BACTERIA

Bacteria are single-celled organisms that grow almost ubiquitously on Earth. They are present in the environment, in the soil and in the water. They are also present in plants and animals, including humans. We all have various species of bacteria living inside our intestinal tract and on our skin. While there are many beneficial species of bacteria, there are also species that are pathogenic and can cause symptoms. While we generally think of being "infected" by a bacteria from an outside source, it is also possible for some of the species that live inside of us, that are usually harmless, to overgrow and cause symptoms. Antibiotics and some other pharmaceuticals can favor this type of bacterial overgrowth.

Causes

1) Airborne
2) Skin contact
3) Water/food contamination
4) Antibiotics and acid-blocker medications (proton-pump inhibitors)
5) Sexual partner (exchange of saliva is enough to pass infection)
6) Pets

Common Symptoms

1) Skin infections
2) Abdominal pain, nausea/vomiting, constipation/diarrhea
3) GERD
4) Respiratory symptoms (rhinitis/sinusitis, sore throat, pneumonia, cough, etc.)
5) Burning, pain with urination
6) Vaginal infections
7) Gingivitis
8) Ear pain/drainage
9) Fatigue

Prevention

1) Filter water
2) Keep the gastrointestinal tract healthy by following a nutrient-dense diet that is low in processed/high-sugar foods, avoiding food allergens/sensitivities, and limiting alcohol consumption.
3) Be as careful as possible with food sources and restaurant choices.
4) If you work in a hospital/doctor's office where you are around sick people, air purifiers can be used to decrease airborne transmission.

5) General hygiene practices such as washing hands before eating, etc.
6) Avoid antibiotic use unless absolutely necessary. If antibiotics must be taken, follow measures to prevent overgrowth of harmful bacteria (i.e. consider taking Morinda Supreme at the same time as the medication and follow up with probiotics, eating cultured foods and possibly taking one of the antimicrobials listed below).
7) Have your partner checked to avoid infection/re-infection.

Supplement Recommendations

SUPREME NUTRITION PRODUCTS

1) Morinda Supreme

2) Melia Supreme

3) Golden Thread Supreme

4) Oral Defense

THORNE RESEARCH

5) Berbercap

6) Isatis

7) Phytogen

8) IM-Encap

9) Olive Leaf Extract

Michael Lebowitz DC and Ami Kapadia MD

Chapter 25:   **HEAVY METALS**

In this chapter, we will be discussing some of the more common metals that can potentially have adverse effects on the body. The metals we will be discussing include: mercury, copper, cadmium, aluminum and lead. This is not an exhaustive list and an alternative health care practitioner can check for these as well as others. For each metal, we will review the sources of exposure and related symptoms. Then, we will discuss general measures that can help to prevent exposure as well as recommendations on reducing your toxic burden if you suspect metal toxicity is contributing to your symptoms.

The question of whether heavy metal toxicity can cause illness in a specific individual depends on several factors. Individuals have widely ranging sensitivities to metals. Therefore, one person may be relatively asymptomatic even after large exposures, while someone who is more sensitive may suffer from various symptoms from much smaller exposures. That is why hair analysis may not be the best indicator (it measures exposure, not sensitivity). In addition, symptoms related to heavy metal toxicity can affect pretty much any organ/body system. We will give you some relatively common symptoms related to toxicity from different metals; however, it is important to keep in mind that "anything can cause anything" when it comes to trying to determine the cause of your symptoms. With heavy metals, there is often a long period, sometimes years, between the time of exposure and the onset of symptoms.

MERCURY

Sources

1) Fish, especially larger fish like tuna, swordfish, shark, tilefish and sea bass (but nearly all fish) are contaminated to some extent. 1 teaspoon of mercury in a 20 acre lake annually renders the fish unsafe to eat.
2) Dental amalgams (also known as "silver" fillings)

3) Mercury containing preservatives that can be found in eye drops and immunizations/vaccines
4) Batteries and thermometers
5) Fungicides (in grains), bactericides and antiseptics
6) Coal burning facilities/power plants
7) Volcanic activity
8) Forest fires
9) Natural deposits
10) Medical waste incineration
11) Fireworks

Symptoms

1) The most common symptom is neurological (any numbness, tingling, loss of balance etc.). It can lead to a named neurological disease or a series of symptoms that don't fit any "textbook definitions" of a specific disease state. Symptoms can be one sided, regional, or body wide.
2) Memory loss and poor recall
3) Birth defects
4) Painful or bleeding gums
5) Unprovoked outbursts of anger or depression
6) Dizziness, impaired speech, in-coordination, and indecision
7) Irritability
8) Excessive salivation and a metallic taste in mouth
9) Fatigue and CFS/FMS
10) Headaches/migraines
11) Visual changes
12) Protein in the urine and sporadic painful urination
13) ADHD/autism spectrum disorders (mercury can contribute to them)

COPPER

Sources

1) Water pipes

2) Algicides for hot tubs/swimming pools etc., fungicides, fertilizers, and insecticides
3) Dyes (hair dye, etc.)
4) Preservatives for leather and fabrics
5) Dental materials (an alloy in gold dental restorations)
6) Cosmetics
7) Fungicide on certain food crops (even organic)
8) Termite treated wood

Symptoms

1) Central nervous system degeneration
2) Disturbed gait, dizziness
3) "Idiopathic" neurological symptoms
4) Immune system, liver and kidney damage
5) Metallic taste
6) Muscle rigidity
7) Nausea/vomiting, constipation/diarrhea, and stomach cramps
8) Psychological impairment
9) Tremors

LEAD

Sources

1) Soil (deposits from leaded gasoline and other environmental sources)
2) Paint in older houses
3) Water pipes
4) Newsprint, ink, ceramics, and paints
5) Electronics
6) Solder
7) Candle wicks
8) Coal burning facilities/power plants
9) Lead painted toys from China, etc.
10) Certain pesticides

Symptoms

1) Lower IQ and memory impairment
2) ADHD/autism spectrum disorders (lead can contribute to them)
3) Impulsive behavior, easy distractibility, and disorganization (especially in kids)
4) Depression, psychosis, irritability, anxiety, and interpersonal conflict
5) Fatigue and weakness
6) Anger and tension
7) Anemia
8) Abdominal pain, nausea/vomiting, diarrhea/constipation and loss of appetite
9) Alterations in sugar and uric acid metabolism
10) Alterations in liver, kidney, thyroid, lung and heart function
11) Convulsions
12) Tremors
13) Visual changes
14) Headaches/migraines

CADMIUM

Sources

1) Food canning
2) Cigarette smoke
3) Coal burning facilities/power plants
4) Asphalt
5) Lime manufacturing
6) Batteries
7) Pigments, paints, and printing
8) Plastics
9) Metal soldering and welding
10) Textiles
11) Contaminated water

Symptoms

1) Hypertension
2) Lung irritation, cough, and emphysema
3) Gastrointestinal irritation, nausea/vomiting, constipation/diarrhea and, abdominal pain
4) Anemia
5) Behavioral problems
6) Cancer (lung and prostate)
7) Contact dermatitis
8) Headaches/migraines
9) Kidney/liver damage
10) Loss of smell
11) Muscle aches and muscle inflexibility
12) Decrease in bone density

ALUMINUM

Sources

1) Antiperspirants
2) Food/drinks in aluminum foil or aluminum cans
3) Some cooking utensils and coatings on pots/pans
4) Antacids and hemorrhoid creams
5) Cosmetics
6) Pharmaceuticals and immunizations used as preservatives.
7) Automotive parts
8) Electrical conductors
9) Food additives (including baking powder)
10) Dental crowns and dentures (porcelain type restorations and some dental composite materials may contain alumina which is aluminum oxide)
11) Paint and protective coatings
12) Fireworks
13) Water purification
14) Sugar refining
15) Rubber and wood preservatives

16) Leather
17) Glues and disinfectants
18) Fiberglass
19) Poor quality supplements and many supplements that have undefined "colloidal" or "ionic" minerals

Symptoms

1) Cough and pulmonary disease
2) Bone diseases
3) Brain dysfunction (linked to dementia and other neurological diseases)
4) Memory loss and poor recall

Treatment/Prevention

Treatment is similar for all forms of metal toxicity. First of all, it is necessary to decrease/remove as many of the current exposures as you possibly can. This would mean avoiding as many of the "sources" (listed under each metal) that are found in your everyday life as possible.

To prevent or treat mercury toxicity, this would mean avoiding seafood (especially fish high in mercury content), not getting additional dental amalgams, and other common sources.

For copper, this would mean using a reverse osmosis water purification system if you have copper pipes and letting your shower or bath water run for a few minutes before stepping in or filling the tub. Avoid copper in cosmetics, hair dye, and dental materials.

For lead, this would mean making sure your home does not have any lead based paint, if it is an older house, and avoiding toys painted with lead based paint.

For cadmium, this would mean avoiding cigarettes and any paints, etc. that contain cadmium.

For aluminum, this would mean avoiding aluminum containing antiperspirants, cosmetics, antacids, baking powder, aluminum-containing pots and pans. Keep aluminum foil out of direct contact with foods and avoid use of foods (especially acidic foods such as tomatoes, orange juice, etc) from aluminum coated cans and drinks in aluminum cans.

In general, to prevent or treat toxic symptoms from metals, or as part of a general metal detoxification program, it is helpful to include sulfur rich foods in the diet as they aid in detoxification. These foods include: Brussels sprouts, onions, garlic, broccoli, cauliflower, kale and eggs. It is generally advised to treat all forms of dysbiosis before (or simultaneously with) starting to detoxify from metals. Please see the dysbiosis chapter for additional information.

Recommended Supplements/medications

The supplements listed below can be helpful for metal detoxification.

SUPREME NUTRITION PRODUCTS

1) Takesumi Supreme

2) Camu Supreme

3) Alaria Supreme

THORNE RESEARCH

4) Captomer (use only under a doctor's supervision)

5) Thiocid

6) Glutathione SR

7) Metaplex

8) Zinc Picolinate

Michael Lebowitz DC and Ami Kapadia MD

Chapter 26: **FOOD ALLERGIES, SENSITIVITIES, AND TOXINS**

It is well known in the holistic medicine world that food reactions can be the cause of various symptoms and illnesses. In this chapter (as we have throughout the book) we will use the terms food allergy, food sensitivity and food intolerance interchangeably to describe a general adverse reaction that a person can have to a food. This is not limited to the traditionally accepted, immediate, IgE type reaction (such as hives, respiratory distress, etc.) that we are all aware of such as an anaphylactic reaction to the ingestion of peanuts. Instead, when we discuss a food allergy in our present context, we will be describing any negative response that a person can have to a given food; it can be immediate or delayed and encompasses symptoms in all body systems.

While it is true that a person can be allergic to virtually any food, we have found that there is a subset of commonly eaten foods that tend to cause most of the trouble. We have identified certain "food toxins" within these common foods that we will discuss; these toxins are either components of the food or proteins found within the food. The potential allergenicity and adverse reactions of these food toxins will be reviewed. Many applied kinesiologists have the Food Toxin Kit (by AK Test Kits) and can test for these types of reactions. Otherwise, total avoidance for 6 weeks followed by re-introduction and observing symptoms is recommended.

ALPHA-SOLANINE ("NIGHTSHADE VEGETABLES")

In the 1950's, Norman F. Childers, a professor of horticulture at Rutgers University, began to investigate the relationship between nightshade plants and arthritic as well as other medical conditions. His work involved examining naturally occurring toxins in food plants. Childers' specific interest in the nightshade group of plants stemmed from his own experience with consumption of members of the *Solanaceae* (or nightshade) family. This group of plants includes: tomatoes, potatoes (except sweet potatoes and yams), eggplant, peppers (all except black and white pepper), paprika, the herb ashwagandha, goji berries and tobacco, as well as other plants that are not generally part of the human diet. Childers noticed that his diverticulitis (condition involving inflammation in the intestinal wall) symptoms, and later his arthritis pain, disappeared when he avoided the nightshade foods. After some of his colleagues and acquaintances had similar relief of chronic symptoms by following the "nightshade-free" diet, Childers decided to recruit volunteers across the country to try his diet.

In 1977, Childers and one of his students, Gerald M. Russo, published the first edition of *The Nightshades and Health*, which describes this association between nightshades and various chronic health ailments such as structural and arthritic type conditions. Childers included numerous abstracts in his book that describe the effects of nightshade plant consumption on livestock such as: gait abnormalities, weakness, osteopetrosis, calcinosis and arterial calcification. He also includes several detailed case reports from the human correspondents who followed his prescribed diet and their experiences involving relief of chronic ailments.

The main compound/chemical thought to be responsible for the potential harmful effects of plants in the nightshade family is alpha-solanine. The amount of solanine present in the above foods varies tremendously depending on growing conditions, time harvested, storage conditions, cooking techniques, etc. Much of the academic work can be credited to Dr. Norman Childers who has been researching nightshades for about 50 years in farm animals, as well as through dietary modification techniques with human correspondents across the country.

Historically, most solanine containing foods were not considered edible before the 1800's (except in some parts of South America). In fact, as late as the 1850's, most Americans considered potatoes a food for animals rather than humans. The Farmer's Manual from that time period recommended that potatoes, "be grown near the hog pens as a convenience towards feeding the hogs." Even foods like kimchee did not have peppers in them 100 years ago and just utilized a salt brine. A few hundred years ago solanine containing foods were mainly used in witchcraft. Now it is rare for people to go a day or even a meal without some form of tomatoes, potatoes, peppers, etc.

Solanines are not water soluble, are not destroyed by cooking and are not broken down inside the body but must be excreted as alpha-solanine. Different people have different degrees of sensitivity to them, and different efficiencies when it comes to excreting them. Solanines can be stored in most organs (with a special affinity for the thyroid gland) as well as most soft tissue including skeletal muscle. How or in what way they will affect you will be a matter of genetics, as well as lifestyle and nutritional status. If you have this problem, the probability is very high that at least one of your parents will have the same condition as there seems to be a genetic link.

Most "foods" that contain alpha-solanine also contain at least 5 other neurotoxins including atropine and nicotine. Acute solanine poisoning can result from ingesting green or sprouted potatoes or green tomatoes, with symptoms including: cramps, nausea, diarrhea, headache, dizziness and sleepiness. In severe cases, partial paralysis and coma can result. However, we are more concerned with "chronic poisoning", which we are calling Solanine Toxicity Syndrome, or STS. STS can result from chronic ingestion of nightshade vegetables in a sensitive individual.

Most of the studies involving the ill-effects of chronic solanine ingestion involve animals. There have been numerous incidences of poisonings in cattle, pigs, sheep and goats feeding on tomato shoots, potato vines, potato peelings and sprouts, and plant tops of several wild species of the nightshade family.

However, Dr. Childers did record the case histories and results that a nightshade free diet had on over 400 correspondents that chose to try it in an attempt to relieve their chronic arthritis (arthritis is one of the many manifestations of STS). The following is a summary of the report issued by Dr. Childers and one of his colleagues:

A total of 434 correspondents returned the questionnaire issued related to the diagnosis of arthritis and their willingness to attempt elimination of nightshades as a form of treatment.

- Of those rigidly on the diet, 94% had complete or substantial relief of symptoms.
- Of dieters with occasional "slips", 50% had complete or substantial relief of symptoms.

- Overall, 68% had complete or substantial relief.

Childers' case histories also emphasized the fact that transgressions in the diet can often result in a recurrence of symptoms.

In addition to resulting in osteoarthritis, on a practical level, it is theorized that nightshades can do the following in sensitive patients:

1) Act as an endocrine disruptor, especially to the thyroid
2) Cause chronic joint pain, all forms of arthritis and joint inflammation
3) Can be a major contributor to arteriosclerosis and osteoporosis
4) Can contribute to "leaky gut", as well as rectal bleeding, IBS, etc.
5) Can contribute to depression
6) Can contribute to migraines
7) Can greatly interfere with calcium and vitamin D absorption, despite supplementation

If you suspect or are found to be sensitive to solanines you need to stay off all nightshades (potato (except for sweet potato/yam), tomato, eggplant, pepper (except for black/white pepper), paprika, tobacco, ashwagandha, and goji berries) for at least 6-8 weeks. Some patients may feel better within days, while it can take months for others to realize the full benefits of avoidance. You should read labels carefully and have 100% avoidance for optimal results (if a label says "spices" and doesn't say what kind, assume it has paprika or red pepper unless you check with the manufacturer). After several weeks to months, if feeling better, try adding back small amounts of nightshades and see how you feel. For many patients, permanent avoidance is necessary to keep symptoms at bay; however, there are patients who can introduce small quantities back into their diet without suffering from a relapse of symptoms.

Personal Observations with Patient Avoidance of Solanines

I had the opportunity to test some professional ballplayers who needed "Tommy John" surgery and they all showed STS. I personally think that STS made them more injury prone. I have seen it test positive on almost all arthritics as well.

In one patient, correcting STS resulted in alleviation of strong suicidal tendencies.

With other patients, it has eliminated post surgical wrist swelling in one, greatly decreased disabling shoulder and neck pain in another (this pain was unresponsive to multiple surgical interventions), eliminated the need for surgery in a patient with chronic bilateral knee pain, eliminated the need for hip replacement surgery in one patient, and resulted in remission in a patient with juvenile rheumatoid arthritis.

I (Dr. Lebowitz) personally experienced a cessation of sporadic rectal bleeding, a greatly increased range of motion in my hip joint, and a 50% decrease in migraine attacks.

Overall, avoidance of solanine containing foods can be a key variable in chronic pain, subluxations, arthritides, any many other chronic symptoms.

Supplement Recommendations

The below may help with Solanine Toxicity Symptoms by helping the body to get rid of solanines faster, but does not fix the underlying sensitivity to solanines.

SUPREME NUTRITION PRODUCTS

> 1) Thera Supreme
>
> 2) Takesumi Supreme

METHYLXANTHINES: CAFFEINE, PARAXANTHINE, THEOBROMINE AND THEOPHYLLINE

Caffeine is the most consumed and socially-acceptable stimulant in the world. Approximately 90% of adults in the world consume caffeine in their daily diet. More than 150 million people in the US drink coffee on a regular basis, averaging 2 cups per day.

Caffeine, as well as theobromine, paraxanthine and theophylline, are part of the methylxanthine family and can be labeled as psychoactive stimulants. These substances in varying amounts and complexes are found in coffee, tea, chocolate, cola, yerba mate and guarana.

Coffee contains caffeine and theophylline, but no theobromine, while tea and chocolate are higher in theobromine. Tea actually contains more caffeine then coffee, but since it is brewed weaker, the average cup of tea has less than the average cup of coffee.

Caffeine Biochemistry and Pharmacokinetics

Caffeine is metabolized in the liver into the following compounds (with approximate percentages): paraxanthine (84%), theobromine (12%) and theophylline (4%).

Caffeine is readily absorbed in the GI tract after oral administration. The average half-life of caffeine is 5 hours (this means that after 5 hours, 50% of the caffeine that you consumed will still be present in your body), with a range of 3-7 hours. Genetic differences in liver detoxification chemistry can be associated with impaired caffeine metabolism and a prolonged half-life (meaning that, in some people, caffeine can take even longer to be broken down).

Symptoms associated with too much caffeine (either too much ingested or impaired breakdown of it) include: headache, anxiety (including generalized anxiety disorder), depression, panic attacks, irritability, tremors, insomnia, nervousness, muscle twitching, increased frequency of spinal subluxations, spinal and joint pain, and GERD.

Using caffeine both short-term and long-term can influence mood and cognition. In addition, heavy coffee intake (>2 cups/day) may trigger coronary and arrhythmic events in susceptible individuals. Finally, it has been shown that excess caffeine consumption (>200 mg/day) during pregnancy may increase the risk of miscarriage.

Theobromine

While theobromine and caffeine are similar, theobromine is a weaker stimulant. Therefore, it can be postulated that theobromine may have a lesser, but still significant, impact on the human central nervous system. While theobromine is not as addictive as caffeine, it has been cited as possibly contributing to chocolate addiction.

Theophylline

In susceptible individuals, theophylline can cause nausea, diarrhea, an increase in heart rate, arrhythmias, and CNS excitation with resultant headaches, insomnia, irritability, dizziness and lightheadedness.

Paraxanthine

Paraxanthine is not produced by plants and is only observed as a metabolite of caffeine in animals/humans. Paraxanthine is the chief metabolite of caffeine breakdown.

Personal Observations

The most common symptoms we see clinically with caffeine sensitivity in our practice are:

1) Locked up joints ("I woke up and my neck won't turn despite having no trauma.")
2) Being prone to musculoskeletal injuries and having them become chronic despite treatment
3) Sleeplessness
4) Anxiety
5) Cardiac symptoms (palpitations, etc)
6) Adrenal weakness (mid afternoon fatigue, postural hypotension, etc)
7) Hemorrhoids and varicose veins

Overall, we have found that a majority (approximately 75%) of patients cannot tolerate the caffeine family. We postulate this is due to the fact that in modern day life the liver is overloaded with environmental toxins, along with generally poor lifestyle factors including a sub-optimal diet, so that caffeine cannot be adequately broken down in most people.

If you suspect the caffeine family is a problem for you (or are found to be sensitive to it), we suggest at least a 1 month avoidance of coffee, tea, yerba mate, chocolate, guarana, acai and cola. There are some remedies that will be listed below that may help accelerate detoxification from caffeine related products; you can consider taking some of these remedies while you are staying off the caffeine family. After the avoidance period, it is possible that you will tolerate caffeine containing foods/beverages in smaller quantities, though some people need long-term avoidance to maintain benefits. Remember it is not uncommon to experience withdrawal symptoms when eliminating caffeine. These can last for up to two weeks.

Supplement Recommendations

The below may help with methylxanthine toxicity symptoms by helping the body to detoxify more easily.

SUPREME NUTRITION PRODUCTS

1. Wild Greens Supreme

2. Body Guard Supreme

3. Reishi Supreme

4. Takesumi Supreme

THORNE RESEARCH

5. Basic B-complex

GLUTEN/GLIADIN

One of the most well publicized food allergens in recent years is gluten. Sensitivity to gluten can cause a wide range of symptoms that can affect almost any organ system. While most would think primarily of Celiac Disease and symptom manifestations in the gastrointestinal tract, the nervous system is actually the second most commonly affected system outside of the gastrointestinal tract and is often involved in sensitive individuals. Some of the symptoms/diagnoses that can be involved with gluten sensitivity include: headaches, behavior changes, seizures, muscle cramps, neuropathy, malnutrition, fatigue, malaise, depression, chronic digestive problems (abdominal pain, diarrhea, constipation, IBS, difficulty gaining/losing weight, reflux, nausea, vomiting, etc.), apthous ulcers, Sjogren's Syndrome, osteoporosis, infertility, miscarriage, thyroid disorders, schizophrenia, autism and dermatitis herpetiformis.

If gluten sensitivity is found, it is necessary to avoid all gluten containing grains, including: barley, rye, wheat, spelt and oats. Oats do not contain gluten but do contain a similar prolamine and many gluten-sensitive people cannot tolerate oats, even if processed in a gluten free facility. It is thus beneficial to avoid oats as well in the beginning of an elimination trial of gluten and then add them in after a few weeks (certified gluten-free types only) and look for symptomatic changes at that time.

CASEIN AND LACTOSE

Casein is one of the main proteins in cow's milk. There is casein in the milk of other species (goat, sheep etc.) of a slightly different nature, and the intolerance can carry over in many sensitive people. Therefore, if a casein sensitivity is suspected, you should avoid all dairy products of all species (many people also react to supposedly casein-free foods like ghee so we avoid these too). Like gluten, casein sensitivity can also cause symptoms in just about any organ system. Specifically, casein sensitivity can contribute to: ear infections, sinus conditions, asthma, eczema, headaches, arthritis, chronic digestive problems, rhinitis, hay fever, depression, mood swings, ADHD, bedwetting and eczema.

Besides having a casein sensitivity, an individual can have a lactose intolerance in which only the gastrointestinal tract is involved (whereas with a casein sensitivity, any organ system can be involved). The main symptoms of lactose intolerance can include bloating, gas, diarrhea, and even vomiting. If this is the case, it is much simpler to address as the patient can simply use lactose-free milk or take a lactase enzyme when consuming dairy products. However, it is important to remember that a lactase enzyme may be a fungal derivative that is not well tolerated.

OVALBUMIN

Ovalbumin is the major protein in egg. In sensitive people, ovalbumin can cause villous atrophy, depletion of mucosal oligosaccharidases, impaired absorption of xylose and depressed serum complement levels. Asthma, as well as most other common symptoms of food intolerance, have been linked to ovalbumin sensitivity. There have even been documented cases of nephropathy that have reversed with egg avoidance. Some vaccines contain albumin in them and we have seen cases of albumin sensitive individuals react to them.

ZEIN

Zein is a class of prolamine protein found in corn. It is also known as corn gluten and even though it too is a prolamine, zein is not chemically identical to wheat or other glutens and the frequency of intolerance is less. Therefore, it can have its own unique effects on the body. Symptoms associated with corn sensitivity can include: headaches, asthma, facial inflammation, rashes, hives, most gastro-intestinal symptoms, fatigue, joint pains and sinus congestion/runny nose, depression.

Personal Observations

Food allergens can be a big part of the puzzle when trying to resolve a wide range of chronic symptoms. We feel that identifying and avoiding allergenic foods can help achieve long-term health and, along with treating dysbiosis and addressing the other root causes that we describe, can help restore the integrity of the gastrointestinal tract.

Once improvement is achieved, some people are able to re-introduce some or all of their allergenic foods in limited quantities without any setbacks, while others need long-term avoidance to remain symptom-free.

Another issue that often comes up is: which came first- the dysbiosis or the food toxin intolerances? It can go in either direction and for optimal results both should be comprehensively addressed.

Supplement Recommendations

The below may be helpful when addressing food allergens (they will not make reactions go away but can lessen the severity of inadvertent ingestions).

SUPREME NUTRITION PRODUCTS

    1. Takesumi Supreme

THORNE RESEARCH

    2. Buffered C Powder

Both these products have lessened the reactions in some individuals. If consumption of allergens cannot be totally avoided, you may want to consider regular supplementation.

Michael Lebowitz DC and Ami Kapadia MD

Chapter 27: NEUROTRANSMITTERS

Neurotransmitters are the chemicals that transmit information or signals from one neuron (nerve cell) to the next in your body. Neurotransmitters are responsible for communication between neurons and can affect a variety of functions including energy levels and mood.

We are going to be discussing three of the main neurotransmitters in the body: epinephrine/norepinephrine, serotonin and GABA.

Catecholamines: Epinephrine and Norepinephrine (and Dopamine)

Epinephrine and norepinephrine make up the class of neurotransmitters called catecholamines. They are excitatory neurotransmitters and help with energy and focus. They are made from an amino acid called tyrosine. Tyrosine can also be converted to dopamine, which has similar functions to catecholamines, and is also known as the pleasure and reward neurotransmitter.

Tyrosine can be depleted by stress, especially emotional stress. Allergies can deplete tyrosine as well (because the body will make more epinephrine to try to deal with allergies). It has been our experience that it is difficult to assimilate tyrosine from food unless you eat a high protein meal without starches/grains. Overall, in clinical experience, we have found that a catecholamine deficiency is actually more common than a serotonin deficiency in patients with depression (sometimes they co-exist, especially when mental imbalances are passed down from one generation to the next and have been relatively severe).

Symptoms of Low Catecholamines/Dopamine

1) Depression with a preference to be left alone
2) Fatigue and low-energy

3) Trouble concentrating, focusing, and a lack of mental sharpness
4) Sleeping a lot and having trouble waking up
5) Decreased libido
6) Dizziness upon rising from sitting/lying down
7) Eyes sensitive to light, especially while driving at night
8) More prone to allergies/sensitivities

Treatment of Low Catecholamines/Dopamine

L-tyrosine in supplement form can be used to normalize levels of catecholamines/dopamine. We would recommend one 500 mg capsule upon awakening and another 500 mg capsule mid-morning (both to be taken seperate from food). We have also found Ashwaganda Supreme to be helpful in normalizing neurotransmitter levels. While it doesn't contain significant amounts of neurotransmitters, it has been shown to normalize neurotransmitter levels. Those with a solanine or nightshade sensitivity (see the food allergy chapter) should not take ashwaganda.

Taking too much tyrosine can sometimes result in too much adrenaline (catecholamines) and cause jitteriness and, in rare cases, elevated blood pressure. In other cases, taking too much can lead to headaches as tyrosine can be converted into tyramine which in susceptible individuals can lead to migraines. All in all it is very safe and one of my most frequently prescribed supplements.

Serotonin

Serotonin has become known as the "happy" neurotransmitter, responsible for a positive mood. Serotonin is necessary in order to maintain a good mood, reduce anxiety/irritability and to help with sleep. Tryptophan is the main amino acid that is needed for your body to make serotonin and is obtained from dietary protein sources. If you eat a low-protein diet, you would be at risk for having low tryptophan and serotonin levels. Other potential causes of low serotonin levels include: stress (causes high cortisol levels which increases the breakdown of tryptophan so less serotonin is made), food allergies/dysbiosis/toxins/high-sugar diet (all cause inflammation and resultant breakdown of tryptophan), a vitamin B6 deficiency (needed to convert tryptophan to serotonin) or a magnesium deficiency.

Symptoms of Low Serotonin

1) Depression with a tendency to want to be around people (rather than being left alone) and tell everyone your "problems"
2) Negative thoughts and low self-esteem
3) Obsessive thoughts and behaviors
4) Irritability, impatience and anxiety
5) Sleep disorders
6) Craving carbohydrates

Treatment of Low Serotonin Levels

Taking the serotonin precursor tryptophan in supplement form as L-tryptophan or 5-hydroxytryptophan (some respond better to one or the other) can help normalize serotonin levels. Our recommended dose for L-tryptophan is one to two 500 mg capsules daily in the evening, seperate from food (typically one an hour after supper and another before bed). The recommended dose of 5-HTP is one to three 50 mg capsules daily in the evening, separate from food (typically one an hour after supper and another before bed).

Note that taking too much L-tryptophan or 5-HTP can leave people feeling groggy the next day. Also, if you are taking prescription medication for depression, you should discuss use of these supplements with your doctor, as combining these supplements with certain medications like SSRIs requires monitoring.

GABA

GABA stands for gamma-aminobutyric acid. It is a neurotransmitter that helps to calm the brain. If this neurotransmitter is low, it becomes difficult for you to relax.

Symptoms of Low GABA

1) Easily stressed out and easily overwhelmed
2) Insomnia
3) Anxiety

Treatment of Low GABA Levels

You can take a GABA supplement to help normalize levels. We recommend THORNE RESEARCH's PharmaGaba 100 mg or PharmaGaba 250 mg. If using the 100's, a recommended starting dose would be 1 capsule twice a day. If using the 250's, a recommended starting dose would be 1 capsule a day in the evening. Many people need double this dose to be effective. Again, take these seperate from food.

Neurotransmitters: General Observations

Neurotransmitter levels can be affected by the different causes discussed above, but can also be out of balance because of a genetic predisposition. Some people are inefficient converters of the raw materials needed to produce the neurotransmitters. The other main root causes of illness that we discuss in this book have a definite impact on mood and can affect neurotransmitter levels. These include: dysbiosis, food allergies, chemical/metal toxicity and nutrient deficiencies. It has been the authors' experience that in patients where the imbalance is not due to a genetic predisposition, supplementation can often be stopped after a certain period of time because neurotransmitter levels normalize after addressing the underlying causes (dysbiosis, food sensitivities, poor dietary habits, etc.).

Some people have multiple neurotransmitter imbalances (e.g. a combination of low catecholamines and low serotonin as mentioned above) rather than just one. For those that suffer from both a catecholamine and serotonin deficiency, it can be helpful to separate protein meals (which are better to eat earlier in the day) from carbohydrate/starch meals (which are better to eat later in the day). This can help with absorption of the raw materials needed for your body to manufacture neurotransmitters. This separation of high starch and high protein meals can also be helpful in people prone to food sensitivities.

It is also helpful to note that serotonin, L-tryptophan (and 5-HTP) and GABA can help with insomnia and sleep disorders in addition to helping with mood. Tryptophan and 5-HTP both can convert to melatonin (which helps with sleep) in addition to converting to serotonin, if the appropriate cofactors are present. Overall cofactors necessary for adequate neurotransmitter production (epinephrine and serotonin) include: B-complex vitamins, magnesium and vitamin C, among others. On some occasions these co-factors need to be supplemented (especially pyridoxal-5-phosphate or B6).

The amino acid precursors to neurotransmitters (tyrosine, tryptophan and 5-HTP) will work better if taken on an empty stomach, either 30 minutes before or 1 hour after a meal.

Cutting out sugar, eating a whole, unrefined foods diet with adequate protein and addressing the root causes of illness will help normalize neurotransmitter levels in the long run. It is also better to eat a higher protein breakfast and lunch and a higher carbohydrate supper to encourage neurotransmitter balance. Prayer, meditation and positive thoughts can all have a positive effect on neurotransmitters as can going to bed early.

Recommended Supplements for Neurotransmitter Rebalancing:

THORNE RESEARCH

    1) L-tyrosine

    2) L-tryptopan

    3) 5-HTP

    5) Pyridoxal-5-Phosphate

SUPREME NUTRITION

    6) Ashwaganda Supreme

Chapter 28: **NUTRITIONAL SUPPLEMENTATION**

I have to admit that I am biased. Over the years, I have worked with supplements from scores of companies and, as a result of blind applied kinesiological comparisons, patient feedback and clinical results, the vast majority of what I prescribe patients comes from 2 companies and you will see recommendations for these products in most chapters. They are listed in each chapter in no particular order as different people's bodies will prefer different ones. You need to use a qualified practitioner or some method of personal biofeedback (muscle testing etc.) to determine which might be best for you. Be forewarned that in the hands of untrained practitioners (and sometimes even trained ones) results of muscle testing and other testing methods can be subjective. But there are many great practitioners out there also. Unlike prescription drugs, side effects are usually very transient and mild for these non prescription items.

The brands I prefer are SUPREME NUTRITION PRODUCTS, THORNE RESEARCH, and LuRONG LIVING.

I have been ordering from THORNE RESEARCH for over 20 years. Their product quality is known throughout the natural health care community. There are vast differences in quality between similar looking supplements due to fillers, binders, dispersing agents, flow agents, solvents used, preservatives, etc. THORNE RESEARCH's emphasis on purity makes it my favorite choice for vitamins, minerals, amino acids, etc. I have been involved with their quality control and formulation to help ensure this as best I can and I am acting as a consultant for them at the time of writing this book.

Supreme Nutrition is a company I helped start. It is a small company with only a handful of products. Each batch of raw materials goes through Applied Kinesiology and clinical testing to assure what we feel is a higher level of quality than just the government required COA's (which, of course, are very important as well). Most of their products are very broad spectrum with health restoration in mind and absolutely no fillers or binders are used in their production.

If you read back issues of my newsletter on my website www.michaellebowitzdc.com you can read scores of case histories of people who responded wonderfully to the techniques we teach and the supplements from these companies.

If you want more information on these products, visit the respective companies' websites or go to my website www.michaellebowitzdc.com where I have write-ups on all the products I use from these companies.

You can order SUPREME NUTRITION PRODUCTS from your natural health care practitioner, by calling 1-800-922-1744, or from their website (www.supremenutritionproducts.com).

You can order THORNE RESEARCH products from your natural health care practitioner. If you do not have a practitioner near you, contact my office for a referral to a physician I have trained or to help you order directly from THORNE RESEARCH (if there is no practitioner in your area). There are many other high quality brands out there, but these two have proven themselves again and again in my work.

A third company I endorse is LURONG LIVING (www.lurongliving.com). This company, like THORNE RESEARCH and SUPREME NUTRITION, has supplements that must meet the highest standards. They have been endorsed by professional athletes in most major sports and can be used by anyone. Their raw materials are evaluated with Applied Kinesiology before being purchased and encapsulated. I suggest visiting their site for more information.

Chapter 29: **ALTERNATIVE HEALTH CARE PHYSICIANS**

Finding a natural physician or alternative medicine physician can be harder than it sounds. They can be DC's, MD's, DO's, ND's, acupuncturists, etc. Oftentimes the license achieved isn't as important as their clinical expertise, philosophy, etc. It is our opinion that if they are trained in some type of feedback system (Applied Kinesiology, electrodermal screening, etc.) these methods can greatly complement a detailed history, lab work, and other tests, to help decide which issues need to be addressed first, what the underlying issues are, and what treatments have the highest possibility of success.

As a chiropractor who specializes in Applied Kinesiology, I have my own personal bias. Applied Kinesiology is a system developed by Dr. George Goodheart back in the 1960's that uses muscle testing as a functional neurological feedback system to help discern what is malfunctioning in the person and what physical and nutritional intervention is needed to help restore the body. I, along with hundreds of thousands of others, are indebted to Dr. George Goodheart for his revolutionary discoveries. The other applied kinesiologist I am most indebted to is Dr. Walter Schmitt, whose unwavering quest for knowledge as well as his genius and humility have stretched and helped make me the physician I am today. Applied Kinesiology is harder than it looks and there are many people who 'muscle test' that are unqualified and subjective in their outcome. This has led to some bad press but a good objective practitioner can get results that appear close to miraculous.

For people who contact me via my website, I am happy to recommend practitioners in your area that I personally know and have trained (if there are any). If I do not know any, I may refer you to the website icakusa.com for names of other applied kinesiologists. The list isn't all inclusive and there are many excellent physicians I am not aware of. You can also encourage one of your practitioners to purchase my training DVD to learn my methods or to attend one of my seminars.

There are other natural healing methods that can be equally helpful so don't give up if there isn't an Applied Kinesiologist near you. Do your homework, ask around, and find a good physician with an open mind who thinks like a detective.

If there is no one, or if it is beyond your budget, utilize the methods in this book. Dr. Kapadia and I may be open to doing phone consultations. Just realize a phone consult is never as good as an in person exam (though Skype does go a long way) and we are acting as nutritional coaches, not doing any diagnosing or treating specific diagnoses since you are not an in person patient. You can contact us via my website if this interests you.

Chapter 30:   **CASE STUDIES**

The case histories here are gleaned from back issues of my free newsletter that goes to approximately 2,000 licensed physicians. You can read more of them on my website www.michaellebowitzdc.com. The ones here are not necessarily the most dramatic but give a broad range of conditions and responses.

At no time do I prescribe prescription medications or make changes in what the patients' physicians prescribed. We also do not make a diagnosis. Based on a careful comprehensive case history, an Applied Kinesiology exam, and 30 years of clinical experience, we try to discern what might be the underlying causes of the patient's symptoms, be it dysbiosis, toxic metals, nutrient imbalances, subclinical endocrine dysfunction, etc. or a combination of these factors. We then make nutritional and dietary recommendations (and sometimes other lifestyle changes), keep in contact with the patient and often do follow-ups every two to three weeks as needed. Again, no diagnosis is made, we do not interfere with traditional medical treatment, and we will refer patients to MD's or DO's as needed. These case histories are from actual patients, some I treated personally and some treated by colleagues of mine who used the same protocols. The patients' names have been changed. Every person is different and not everyone with the same symptoms will respond to the same diet and supplements. Being a chiropractor, I also addressed their musculo-skeletal misalignments which may very well have enhanced the results. Some patients respond very quickly, some slower and a few not at all. Some of these come in the form of testimonials written by the patients themselves.

Read them to see how important dysbiosis, food reactions, toxic metals, and proper supplementation can be. I tried to pick some from each category but, as you will see, many people have a number of findings in each category that should ideally all be addressed. We do not claim to have cured anyone but are reporting the patients' subjective opinions on their improvement.

Case Study #1

"For about three months, our five-year-old daughter, Alexandra, had been experiencing stomach discomfort after eating. Plain vegetables, rice, and in the end, even water seemed to disturb her intestines. Her energy dissipated and she began to dread meal-times. Desperate for relief for our daughter, we brought her to see Dr. Lebowitz. Within moments, Dr. Lebowitz was able to diagnose the source of the discomfort as a wheat allergy accompanied by possible fungal involvement. Morinda Supreme powder was recommended for treatment. Within days, Alexandra was able to eat normally. Her appetite returned and the dark circles that had begun to dominate her bright face disappeared within a week. Once again, thanks to Dr. Lebowitz and the Morinda Supreme powder, our vibrant young daughter is once again singing and dancing around our home."

Case Study #2   (from a practitioner in Sweden)

I still get amazed by how wonderful this work is and what influence some things can have on a body. Today we checked a 3 month old baby (from England), who has cried all the time she was awake since birth. She is breast fed, but gets some food too. During the checkup, we found evidence of dysbiosis. We prescribed Morinda Supreme. We also found intolerance to some foods: potato, sweet potato, rice, gluten, wheat and oat. He also tested badly on breast milk. He was screaming all the time... We desensitized. After that he fell asleep and we did a checkup on his mother. When he woke up again, he didn't cry for the first time since birth and neither did he cry for the rest of the time during their visit. He even looked more calm and harmonious. The mother was amazed and could not believe it!

Case Study #3

I just received a letter from 2 patients I first saw in March (a married couple). Marion is 54. Wes is 50. Marion came in with a TSH of 5.19

(normal being 0.4-4.0, she had thyroid cancer in 1983) and a total cholesterol of 240. She was relatively asymptomatic from a symptom standpoint. Marion writes "Wes and I are so very "grateful" to G-d to have you so nearby for health needs, you are such a blessing. My amazing health miracle, and then Wes called a day after his appointment with you to say he has not felt this good in years! Thank you."

In our exam of Marion we found sensitivities to potato and garlic. We also strongly suspected dysbiosis. We supplemented with Artecin, Basic B-complex, Biomins II, and L-Tyrosine (THORNE RESEARCH). She returned 6 weeks later to report her total cholesterol had dropped to 181 (LDL went from 175 to 120), and her TSH dropped to 3.07. We dropped the Artecin at that point but continued the others. Her husband just basically needed some good general Applied Kinesiological treatment and supplementation with PicMins (THORNE RESEARCH).

Case Study #4

Chris is a 33-year-old male who first came in April with a chronic severe case of eczema. He used topical steroids for many years and was recently changed to Eladil (a different type of immune suppressant). He also had a cold of 6 weeks duration and athletes foot continuously since 1990. We strongly suspected dysbiosis (especially fungal) and sensitivities to peanut, egg and wheat. He also needed Coconut Oil Supreme, Morinda Supreme (SUPREME NUTRITION) and Zinc Carbonate (THORNE RESEARCH). We desensitized him, had him temporarily avoid the foods and took him off refined sweetening and fermented foods. Chris returned 18 days later with about 80% improvement. We kept him on the supplements and his condition eventually resolved.

Case Study #5   (from a physician friend)

'I had a 50-year-old female diagnosed with Crohn's Disease last year come in with the usual complaints associated with the disorder. She was nicknamed "20 minute Donna" by her office staff because she would be headed for the bathroom within that time after every meal. The excessive diarrhea would make her extremely weak and then she would pass out. She also complained of headaches and fatigue. We strongly suspected dysbiosis and sensitivities to garlic and tuna. We supplemented with SF722, Artecin, Isatis, Citramins, Basic B and 5HTP (THORNE RESEARCH).

She came in for her 3 week check-up and stated that she has had just "normal" daily bowel movements for the last two weeks and feels wonderful. She was cleared of dysbiosis but needed to continue the Citramins and Basic B.

Case Study #6

Bonnie is an 18-year-old who owns her own successful clothing store. When she graduated high school she was all set up to pursue a career in professional modeling in New York City. For no apparent reason, since graduation she was plagued with panic attacks on a daily basis along with many fears. She had been a very friendly outgoing person but now she couldn't drive (due to fear) and had a hard time being around people. She also started suffering from postural hypotension, dizziness with neck extension, brain fog, fatigue, chronic yeast infections, PMS, as well as a 10 pound weight gain. We suspected dysbiosis and sensitivities to tuna, lamb, potato, and tomato. We desensitized her and placed her on the following supplements: SF722 (which we placed her boyfriend on too), Basic Nutrients V and L-Tyrosine (all THORNE RESEARCH). We took her off the 4 foods she was sensitive to (she cheated once, ate a potato, and broke out in a rash as a result), along with all sweetening and fermented food. Bonnie returned for a follow up 3 weeks later. She reported that she no longer had panic attacks (in fact she just returned from a car trip to LA, which required many contacts with business people). She no longer was dizzy, had greatly increased energy and had lost eight pounds. Basically she was her "old" self again. On retesting with Applied Kinesiology, all the initial findings were negative, though we had to keep her on L-Tyrosine and Basic Nutrients V.

Case Study #7

The Carter family came to see me in October. In 1998 they moved into a house, unaware that it was heavily infested with "rhizo mucor", a toxic fungus. Over the next year Tim, age 41, and his wife Bertha, age 32, developed severe joint pains, brain fog and fatigue. Tim also developed dermatitis, chronic headaches, weak knees, and had gained 30 pounds for no apparent reason. He became too disabled to work. Bertha developed "lung problems", chronic flu like symptoms, diarrhea and chronic severe headaches. The doctors were unable to diagnose them and put them both on prednisone.

Mickey, their son, now 10, had been suffering since then with frequent spontaneous nose bleeds and became highly irritable and emotional. Kelly, now 8, became a bed wetter and suffered from a very poor memory even forgetting how to buckle a seatbelt. Noah, now 4, was born in that house, threw frequent tantrums and had chronic constipation.

In 2002 they moved out of the house after the mold problem was discovered and had minor improvement, but with the organisms still living inside them, it wasn't nearly enough. They heard about us this fall and booked an appointment for the whole family. We suspected fungal problems in all 5 but no other forms of dysbiosis. Each had 2 or 3 food sensitivities except Noah, who had six (this was our educated guess based on Applied Kinesiology testing). They all tested for SF722 and Basic Nutrients I and Bertha also needed Thiocid (all by THORNE RESEARCH).

We rechecked them one month later. Tim and Bertha no longer had joint pain and within 3 days of starting the program Tim could raise his arm over his head (this is with no structural treatment). He hadn't been able to perform that motion for over 5 years. He was headache free, dermatitis free, had 75% memory improvement, and was well enough to begin looking for work. Bertha was now asymptomatic. The children's emotional outbursts had ceased and their memories had improved tremendously. Noah was no longer constipated. Mickey no longer had any nosebleeds. Kelly no longer had any bedwetting.

Because they were mainly suffering from fungal dysbiosis, were no longer living in a moldy house, and were compliant patients, they all responded quickly. It was an extremely satisfying case. I only wish I had seen them four years earlier to decrease the time they suffered. I also feel they all had strong constitutions; otherwise our findings would have been much more extensive.

Case Study #8

Tammi is a 36-year-old female who has suffered from severe anxiety problems for 7 years. It started post partum and after a move to a moldy house. It had been fairly disabling, but she couldn't take prescription medicine due to the side effects. Our exam was suggestive of dysbiosis and a neurotransmitter imbalance. We desensitized her, took her off refined sweetening and fermented foods for 14 days and supplemented with Morinda Supreme (SUPREME NUTRITION), L-Taurine, L-Tyrosine (1 on awakening, 1 mid-morning) and 5 HTP (1 early evening and 1 before bed) (THORNE RESEARCH). She returned 3 weeks later (she lives a 6 hour drive away) to report that she was symptom free for the first time in seven years. We kept her on the supplements and continue to monitor her.

Case Study #9

Bobby is a 48-year-old male who was "poisoned" by malathion over a decade ago. Since then he has suffered from low back pain, fatigue, a very short temper, bad body odor and dark circles under his eyes. Besides pesticide poisoning, we suspected sensitivities to beef and garlic. We supplemented with Body Guard Supreme, Endo Supreme and Takesumi Supreme (SUPREME NUTRITION) as well as L-Tyrosine, and PharmaGaba (THORNE RESEARCH). Within a month Bobby was symptom free and very happy. He is staying on maintenance doses of Takesumi and Body Guard.

Case Study #10

Stevie is a 4-year-old asthmatic. The condition has been going on for 2 years and twice a year he contracts pneumonia. He uses albuterol as needed. We suspected multiple forms of dysbiosis (our case history brought out the fact that his bathroom was moldy). He also appeared sensitive to rice, egg, chocolate, wheat, olive, cherry, vinegar and turkey. The only supplement we gave him was Morinda Supreme. We put him on the appropriate diet and had his parents clean his bathroom with tea tree oil, water and borax. We rechecked him 5 weeks later (he lives 4 hours away). He has not had any symptoms of asthma since 5 days after the treatment started and we (as well as his family physician) continue to monitor him.

Case Study #11   (from a colleague)

A patient came in three weeks ago today. For three months he had a "rash" on his chest, genitals, and groin. I saw that it was fungal in nature (ringworm and probably more). He has had digestive problems for years. He complained of problems eating anything without pain. He has had acupuncture since and that helped. I put him on the following: Morinda Supreme, Takesumi Supreme, Alaria Supreme, Endo Supreme (SUPREME NUTRITION), Basic Nutrients III and Omega Plus (THORNE RESEARCH)

Today he came in and the "rash" on his chest, groin and genitals is totally gone. If he eats a big steak, pork and sometimes bananas he still gets a "burning" sensation in his gut and sometimes under his tongue. We continued him on Morinda Supreme and added Betaine HCl (THORNE RESEARCH) and he continues to do well.

Case Study #12

Karen is a 17-year-old high school student. Six weeks before her appointment she had a week of on and off vomiting that stopped but left her with unremitting severe abdominal pain in the area of her spleen, as well as exhaustion and severe headaches. Her bowels were normal. She was finishing up a 90 day course of Solodyn (minocycline) for acne when this happened. The pain was not getting better. She had undergone upper and lower GI's that were negative, blood work was negative and a gynecological exam was negative. The physicians said birth control pills would be the next step.

According to the PDR, possible GI side effects from Solodyn included enterocolitis, pancreatitis, hepatitis, and liver failure.

We suspected multiple forms of dysbiosis and supplemented with Morinda Supreme, Melia Supreme, Takesumi Supreme and Body Guard Supreme (SUPREME NUTRITION). We scheduled her for a follow-up in 14 days. Karen reported she was 98% pain free (a slow steady improvement over 14 days) and her energy was 98% back to normal. Our re-exam showed no findings at this point. We kept her on Melia Supreme and Takesumi Supreme and we (and her family physician) continue to monitor her as needed. Needless to say, she and her mom were very pleased.

Case Study #13

Hank is a 74-year-old man who spent over a decade working in China setting up factories. In many of his locations the pollution was so bad that "you couldn't see the sun because of the air quality". He was seeing an osteopath in his home town, which is about 2 hours away, who was unable to help him and gave him the option of going to the Mayo Clinic or to me. Being more naturally oriented, he chose to see me first. Dr. Kapadia and I worked together on Hank. When he first arrived he needed help walking (a cane) due to his unsteady gait. He also fell "quite often". This had been going on for 8 months and progressing. Both legs were extremely swollen, painful, red, and hot and he was diagnosed with prostate cancer with a PSA of 21. He opted against surgery and radiation and decided to let it runs its course. He came to me due to his balance/gait issues. He also occasionally had a metallic odor to him. Our initial exam suggested multiple forms of dysbiosis, intolerance to methylxanthines, casein, gliadin, ovalbumin (egg), alpha-solanine, and toxicity to mercury.

We took him off the positive food toxins and gave him the following supplements: Captomer 250 (1-2x/day), Methylcobalamin (1x/day) (THORNE RESEARCH); Morinda Supreme (3x/day), Oral Defense (1 drop rubbed on gums before and after brushing teeth), Takesumi Supreme (1 scoop 2x/day), and Camu Supreme (1 scoop 2x/day) (SUPREME NUTRITION PRODUCTS).

Hank was very compliant and returned in 3 weeks. His pain and swelling had decreased about 70% and he no longer needed a cane to walk. We looked more closely at metals and testing suggested problems with mercury, copper, platinum, gold, iron, nickel, lead, thallium and beryllium. His dysbiosis was resolved. Because he was 100% compliant, the food toxins did not test positive but we felt it was premature to try re-introducing the foods to his diet. He continued on the diet. We dropped Oral Defense and Methyl Cobalamine and added Gluathione SR and L-Tyrosine (THORNE RESEARCH). The rest of the supplements stayed the same.

We saw Hank again in 5 weeks. His legs were now normal; no pain, redness, or swelling. Supplements stayed the same. A month later he had a spryness in his step like a 20 year old. Aluminum and lead were added to the findings (as you chelate metals out it is not unusual to see new ones on testing as they come "out of storage").

We had him re-introduce small amounts of the food toxins before coming in last week to see how sensitive his body was to them. Only the methylxanthines tested positive which meant he could tolerate the others at least at the twice weekly amounts we had him experiment with. We will have him increase these to see if he can handle more (but no methylxanthines at all). His supplementation stays steady (Captomer 250, Glutathione SR, Takesumi, Camu) except we were able to drop the Tyrosine. He still has some dizziness at times but it doesn't affect his gait. I feel like he has his life back. His PSA has dropped from 21 to 14 without any medical treatment directed at it, which has been an added bonus we did not expect as we did nothing directly to treat that condition. We continue to see him approximately once a month. He stays on Captomer, Takesumi and now takes Wild Greens Supreme by SUPREME NUTRITION PRODUCTS.

Hank is a pleasure to work with. At 72, I had no idea if we could help or not but he has responded well.

Case Study #14

Steven is a 24-year-old male. He had been diagnosed with juvenile rheumatoid arthritis at age 15 and ulcerative colitis at 16. He had been on Prednisone for 4 years and then Remicade for 4 years. Each only gave him minor improvement and he decided to look for an alternative when he started having major side effects from the medications. He also had athletes foot, fatigue and suffered from migraines (2-3x/week).

Our exam and his history suggested fungal involvement as well as problems with solanines, casein and methylxanthines. We took him off the suspect foods and gave him Morinda Supreme, Takesumi Supreme, and LuRong (SUPREME NUTRITION). Steven became asymptomatic within 2 weeks. He found that when he "cheated by eating potatoes" his RA would flare up. Being a young man, he is contemplating if a life without these foods is worth being pain free. He knows cause and effect in this case. I feel it is my job to find the underlying cause and demonstrate it to the patient and then the decisions are up to him/her.

REFERENCES:

1. "How Much Vitamin D is Too Much?", Med. World News pg. 100-103 1/13/75

2. "Self Styling and the Thymus", Science News Vol. 113, No. 12 pg. 186

3. Airola, P *How to Get Well* Health Plus Publishers, Phoenix, 1974

4. Airola, P *Everywoman's Book* Health Plus Pub., Phoenix, 1979

5. Altschul, R. and Heima, I.H. "Ultraviolet and Cholesterol Metabolism", Circ 8:438 1953

6. Baker S. *Detoxification and Healing*. Revised Edition. McGraw-Hill; 2004.

7. Baldwin, B. "The Pituitary", Journal of Health and Healing Vol. 8 No. 3 1983 pg. 6-8

8. Barnes, Broda and Galton, L. *Hypothyroidism: The Unsuspected Illness* T.Y. Corwell, N.Y. 1976

9. Beardall, Alan *Clinical Kinesiology Instruction Manual* Clinical Kinesiology, Lake Oswego, Oregon 1982

10. Beardall, Alan *Clinical Kinesiology Vol* 1-4

11. Bellet, S. et al. "Effect of Caffeine on Ventricular Fibrillation Threshold", Amer. Heart Journal 54: 215-227 1972

12. Bierenbaum, M. et al. Circ. 42:943 1970

13. Broderick P, Benjamin AB. Caffeine and psychiatric symptoms: a review. J Okla State Med Assoc. 2004; 97 (12):538-42.

14. Burton, A.C. *Physiology and Biophysics of the Circulation* Yearbook Med. Pub. Inc., Chicago 1965

15. Cannon ME, Cooke CT, McCarthy JS. Caffeine-induced cardiac arrhythmia: an unrecognized danger of healthfood products. Med J Aust 2001; 174: 520-1.

16. Carrillo JA, Benitez J. CYP1A2 activity, gender and smoking, as variables influencing the toxicity of caffeine. Br J Clin Pharmacol 1996; 41: 605-608.

17. Chapman, F. *An Endocrine Interpretation of Chapman's Reflexes* Amer. Acad. Of Osteopathy, Colorado Springs 1963

18. Childers, NF, Russo, GM. *The Nightshades and Health.* 1st Ed. Somerville, New Jersey: Somerset Press, Inc.; 1977.

19. Chopra A, Morrison L. Resolution of caffeine-induced complex dysrhythmia with procainamide therapy. J Emerg Med 1995; 13:113-117.

20. Christopher, John *School of Natural Healing* Bi World Pub., Provo, Utah 1976

21. Clemente, C. *Anatomy, A Regional Atlas of The Human Body* Lea and Febiger, Philadelphia, 1975

22. Cornelis MC, El-Sohemy A, Kaagambe EK, Campos H. Coffee, CYP1A2 genotype, and risk of myocardial infarction. JAMA 2006; 295: 1135-1141.

23. Cremer, R.J. et al. "Influence of Light on the Hyperbilirubinemia in Infants", Lancet 1:1227 1958

24. Davidek, J, editor. *Natural Toxic Compounds of Foods, Formation and Change During Food Processing and Storage.* Boca Raton, Florida: CRC Press; 1995.

25. Delamere, J.P., Scott. D.L., et al. "Thyroid Dysfunction and Rheumatic Diseases", JR Soc. Med 75: 102-106, 1982

26. Dennison, Paul *Switching On* Edukinesthetics Inc., Glendale, Calif. 1981

27. Devries, Julian "Contraceptive Pill Criticized", Arizona Republic 8/7/75

28. Diamond, J. *Your Body Doesn't Lie* Warner Books, N.Y. 1979

29. Field, Sidney, Readers Digest Feb. 1976

30. Fowler, M. *Nightshade Free Pain Free!* Michael Fowler; 2007.

31. Frank, C.W. et al. "Physical Activity as a Lethal Factor in Myocardial Infarction Among Men", Circulation 34: 1022 1966

32. Fredholm BB, Battig K, Holmen J, Nehlig A, Zvartau EE. Actions of caffeine in the brain with special reference to factors that contribute to its widespread use. Pharmacol Rev 1999: 51; 83-133.

33. Friedman, M. et al. J.A.M.A. 193:882 1965

34. Galland L, Barrie S. Intestinal dysbiosis and the causes of disease. J. Advancement Med. 1993; 6: 67-82.

35. Galland L. *The Four Pillars of Healing*. New York: Random House; 1997.

36. Garner, C. *Special Techniques of Applied Kinesiology* Clifford Garner, Santa Clara, Calif. 1983

37. Getz, G.S. et al. "Lipids in Rhesus Monkeys", Circ. Supplement 2 35:11-13 1967

38. Giardina E. Cardiovascular effects of caffeine. http://uptdol.com. 2009.

39. Goodheart, G. *Applied Kinesiology Workshop Procedure Manual 1981-1983* G. Goodheart Inc., Detroit 1983

40. Guyton A. *Basic Human Physiology* WB Saunders, Philadelphia, 1977

41. Hadjivassiliou A, Chattopadhyay A, Davies-Jones G, et al. Neuromuscular disorder as a presenting feature of coeliac disease. J Neurol Neurosurg Psychiatry 1997: 63; 770-775.

42. Hansen, R. *Get Well At Home* The College Press, Collegedale, Tennessee 1980

43. Hoffman, Jay M. *The Missing Link* Prof. Press Pub Co., Valley Center, Cal. 1981

44. Honda, Y. et al. "Growth Hormone Secretion During Nocturnal Sleep in Normal Subjects", J. Clin. Endo. Metab. 29:20-29 1969

45. Huggins C "Endocrine Factors in Cancer", J. Urology 68:857 1952

46. Hyman M. *The Ultramind Solution*. New York NY: Scribner; 2009.

47. Johnson, Gomes, and Vandemark *The Testes Vol. 3* Academic Press, New York, 1970

48. Kabagambe EK, Wellons MF. Benefits and risks of caffeine and caffeinated beverages. http://utdol.com. 2009.

49. Kadans, J. *Modern Encyclopedia of Herbs* Parker Pub, W. Nyack, N.Y. 1970

50. Kapit, W. and Elson, L. *The Anatomy Coloring Book* Harper and Row, N.Y. 1977

51. Kime, Z. *Sunlight could Save your Life* World Health Pub., Pennyn, Cal. 1980

52. Leonard, J., Hofer, J., and Pritikin, N. *Live Longer Now* Grosset and Dunlap, N.Y. 1974

53. Mae, E. *How I Conquered Cancer Naturally* Harvest House, 1975

54. Magoun, Harold *Osteopathy In The Cranial Field* Sutherland Cranial Teaching Foundation, Meridian, Ohio 1976

55. Malterre T, Malterre A. *The Whole Life Nutrition Cookbook.* 2nd Ed. Bellingham, WA: Whole Life Press; 2008.

56. Menon, I.S. et al. "Effects of Strenuous Exercise and Graded Exercise on Fibrinolytic Activity", Lancet 700 4/1/67

57. Moore, R., et al. "Central Control of the Pineal Gland: Visual Pathways", Archives Neurology 18:208-218 1968

58. Morrison, L.M. "Diet in Coronary Atherosclerosis", J.A.M.A. 173:884-888 1960

59. Myerson and Neustaldt "Influence of Ultraviolet Light Irradiation Upon Excretion of Sex Hormones in the Male", Endocrinology 25:7 1930

60. Netter, Frank *CIBA Collection Vol.1 The Nervous System* CIBA, Summit, N.J. 1972

61. Osman, Betty *Learning Disabilities A Family Affair* Random House, N.Y. 1979

62. Ott, John *Light, Radiation and You* Devin-Adair Co., Old Greenwich, Conn. 1982

63. Ott, John *Health and Light* Simon and Schuster, N.Y. 1973

64. Parker, D.C. et al. "Human Growth Hormone Release During Sleep, EEG Correlation", J. Clin. Endo. Metab. 29: 871-874 1969

65. Peterson, S. *Hydrotherapy in the Home* Eden Valley Inst., Loveland, Col. 1973

66. *Physician's Desk Reference* Med. Eco. Co. Oradell, N.H. various editions

67. Poesnecker, G.E. *Its Only Natural* Ad Ventures Ltd. Lansdale, Pa. 1975

68. Potera, Carol "The Two Faces of Aspirin", Your Life and Health, Sept. 82

69. Revkin, Andrew "Paraquat, A Potential Weed Killer is Killing People", Science Digest June 1983

70. Rossiter, F. *Water for Health and Healing* HC White Pub., Riverside, Cal 1972

71. Schalch, D.S. "The Influence of Physical Stress and Exercise on Growth Hormone and Insulin Secretion in Man", J. Lab. Clin. Med. 68:256 1963

72. Scheer, J. "Solved the Riddle of Heart Attacks", Let's Live Apr. 77 pg. 56-64

73. Schmitt, W. *Common Glandular Dysfunction in the General Practice* Applied Kinesiology Study Program, Chapel Hill, N.C. 1981

74. Shamberger, R., Journal of National Cancer Institute May 1971

75. Stoner, Fred *The Eclectic Approach to Chiropractic* FLS Pub. Co., Las Vegas 1975

76. Sutton, R.B. et al. "The Hormonal Response to Physical Exercise", Aust. Ann. Med 18: 84 1969

77. Taylor, A. et al. "Electrophysiological Evidence for the Action of Light on The Pineal Gland in the Rat", Exper. 26:267 1970

78. *The Merck Manual* ,Merck Sharp and Dohme, Rahway, N.J. various editions

79. *The New Layman's Parallel Bible* Zondervan Bible Pub., Grand Rapids, Mich. 1981

80. Thie, John *Touch for Health* De Vorsse Co., Marina del Rey, Cal. 1973

81. Thomas, W. et al. American Journal of Cardiology Jan. 1960

82. Thrash, A. and Thrash, C. *Natural Remedies* Yuchi Pines Inst., Seale, Alabama 1983

83. Thrash, A. and Thrash, C. *Home Remedies* Yuchi Pines Inst., Seale, Alabama 1981

84. Thrash, A. and Thrash, C. *Health Counseling Reference Library* Yuchi Pines Inst., Seale, Alabama

85. Travell, J. and Simmons, D. *Myofascial Pain and Dysfunction* Williams and Wilkin, Baltimore/London 1983

86. Vendon, Shirley *Food for the Whole Man Health Seminar Enrichment Course* Shirley Vendon, Deer Park, Cal.

87. Walther, David *Applied Kinesiology Programmed Instruction* Systems DC, Pueblo, Colorado, 1977

88. Walther, D. *Applied Kinesiology, The Advanced Approach to Chiropractic* Systems DC. Pueblo, Col. 1976

89. Walther, David *Applied Kinesiology Vol 1 and 2* Systems DC, Pueblo, Colorado 1981, 1982

90. Weng X, Odouli R, D-K Li. Maternal caffeine consumption during pregnancy and the risk of miscarriage: a prospective cohort study. A J Obstet Gynecol 2008; 198: 279.e1-279.e8.

91. West. S. *Golden Seven Plus One* Samuel Publishing, Orem, Utah 1981

92. Wetterberg L. et al. "Harderian Gland: An Extraretinal Photoreceptor Influencing the Pineal gland in Neonatal Rats?", Sci. 167: 884-5 1970

93. Wilson C. *Chemical Exposure and Human Health: A Reference to 314 Chemicals with a Guide to Symptoms and a Directory of Organizations.* Jefferson, North Carolina: McFarland and Company, Inc.; 1993.

94. Winter, Ruth *A Consumer's Guide to Food Additives* Crown Publishers, N.Y. 1972

95. Wolfsen, Al *Healing By God's Natural Methods* Pirapo, Paraguay 1972

96. Wright, M. *Practical Home Healing* Destiny Press, Queensland, Australia

97. Wurtman, R. "The Pineal and Endocrine Function", Hospital Practice Vol. 4 No. 1 pg. 32-7 1968

98. Wurtman, R. et al. "Environmental Lighting and Neuroendocrine Function: Relationship between Spectrum of Light Source and Gonadal Growth", Endo 85:1218-1221 1969

For further reading on hypoallergenic diets and elimination diets with recipes, I would suggest the following book:

Soon to be released: The Body Restoration Cookbook

Health Care Practitioners can get further information and subscribe to my free newsletter by going to: www.michaellebowitzdc.com